Contemporary Occupational Health Nursing

A guide for practitioners

Edited by Greta Thornbory

Written by and on behalf of the Association of Occupational
Health Nurse Practitioners (AOHNP)

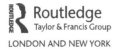

Routledge
Taylor & Francis Group

LONDON AND NEW YORK

First published 2014
by Routledge
2 Park Square, Milton Park, Abingdon, Oxon, OX14 4RN

and by Routledge
711 Third Avenue, New York, NY 10017

*Routledge is an imprint of the Taylor & Francis Group, an informa
business*

British Library Cataloguing in Publication Data
A catalogue record for this book is available from the British Library

Library of Congress Cataloging in Publication Data
  Contemporary occupational health nursing: a guide for practitioners/
  edited by Greta Thornbory
      p.; cm
  1. Thornbory, Greta, editor of compilation. II. Association of
  Occupational Health Nurse Practitioners, issuing body.
  [DNLM: 1. Occupational Health Nursing—Great Britain. WY 141]
  RC966
  610.73'46—dc23   2013021785

ISBN: 978-0-415-82294-7 (hbk)
ISBN: 978-0-415-82295-4 (pbk)
ISBN: 978-0-203-55302-2 (ebk)

Typeset in Sabon
by Swales & Willis Ltd, Exeter, Devon

The Association of Occupational Health Nurse Practitioners (UK) wishes to dedicate this book to the memory of Dorothy Radwanski FRCN (1928–2012), pioneer in occupational health nurse education and first chief nurse to the Health and Safety Executive 1974–1983

Contents

Figures

Tables

Boxes

Contributors

Christina Butterworth
RGN SCPHN-OH Dip OH PG Dip HEHP
President, AOHNP (UK)
Head of Health, BG Group

Siân Edwards
MSc RN(Adult) Dip OH TechIOSH
South West Regional Director AOHNP (UK)
Independent OH Advisor

Susanna Everton
MSc RGN SCPHN-OH CSP CMIOSH
London Regional Director AOHNP (UK)
OH and Safety Practitioner

Anna Harrington
BSc(Hons) RGN
Midlands Region Director AOHNP (UK)
OH Nurse specialising in wellbeing and mental health

Teresa Harrison
BSc(Hons) RGN SCPHN-OH DMS
Vice President
AOHNP (UK)
OH Manager, Leicestershire Fire and Rescue Service/Forge Health

Kate Kyne
MBA RGN SCPHN-OH, DipOHN
Director AOHNP (UK)
NHS
Head of OH and Wellbeing. Great Western Hospitals NHS Foundation Trust

Sarah Mogford
MSc BSc(Hons) RGN CMIOSH
NE and East Anglia Regional Director AOHNP (UK)
Specialist OH Practitioner

Andy Phillips
BSc(Hons) OH, RN (Adult) SCPHN-OH
Wales and International Director AOHNP (UK)
OH Nurse; Director: Eminence Occupational Health and Lecturer/practitioner: University
    of South Wales

Diane Romano-Woodward
M Med Sc(OH) BSc RN SCPHN-OH
Research advisor to AOHNP (UK)
Director, Sunny Blue Sky Limited

Jeremy Smith
BSc(Hons) (OHN) RGN SCPHN-OH
Dip Coach Dip NLP Dip Hypnosis
Past President AOHNP (UK)
Independent OH Consultant and Business Health Coach

Greta Thornbory
MSc RGN SCPHN-OH
DipNOH PGCEA
Professional Development Director AOHNP (UK)
Consultant OH Nurse

Foreword

The professions engaged in the provision of occupational health (OH) services have experienced major changes in the last ten years. Research has demonstrated that good work is good for health, and based on that premise, Dame Carol Black's recommendations in 2008 in *Working for a Healthier Tomorrow*[1] have led to a greater emphasis on the need for support and rehabilitation for workers in the workplace. In 2012 the government announced its intention to set up an Independent Advisory and Assessment Service, staffed by qualified OH professionals, taking over the certification of fitness for work from general practitioners after 4 weeks' sickness absence.

OH is fast becoming a multidisciplinary service, and this has been reflected in the creation of the Council for Work and Health, bringing together doctors, nurses, physiotherapists, psychologists, ergonomists, health and safety practitioners and others with the aim of working together and speaking with one voice. Many OH services are managed by senior nurses, so that management skills are now required in addition to technical competence in monitoring and advising on work-related health. The decline of heavy industry and the rise of modern working methods, such as computing and telesales, have created new workplace hazards. There is an increasing need to justify health interventions by evidence-based research.

These developments have cast doubt on the historical categorisation of OH nurses by the Nursing and Midwifery Council as public health nurses in the same group as school nurses and health visitors. As OH becomes more specialised, the need for training in, for example, health surveillance and case management and rehabilitation increasingly has to be provided by courses which are not validated by the Nursing and Midwifery Council. This book seeks to provide a highly practical guide for OH nurses. It is written by specialists in the field and reflects the skills which are needed to provide an efficient OH service in the second decade of the twenty-first century.

Professor Diana Kloss
Chair, Council for Work and Health
May 2013

Reference

1 Black C (2008) *Working for a Healthier Tomorrow*. London: TSO. Available online at: http://www.dwp.gov.uk/docs/hwwb-working-for-a-healthier-tomorrow.pdf (accessed 09.01.13).

Preface

Occupational health (OH) nursing is a specialist branch of public health nursing requiring specific knowledge and skills. It differs from all other branches of public health nursing as it is concerned with the health of people at work and the effects of work on health and health on work. This area of healthcare has long been in the shadows but the acknowledgement of its importance to the UK economy has been highlighted to recent governments in reports by the Work Foundation, Dame Carol Black and other eminent organisations and health professionals, all of whom will be discussed within the text. Since the publication of these works, OH is at the forefront of healthcare today as the UK government has realised the economic need for people to be and remain in work throughout their life. OH nurses are in the front line, delivering health advice to the working population, advising management and striving to improve the health and wellbeing of the adult population.

Specialist education and training are required to prepare the qualified and registered nurse to undertake OH nursing. The aim of this book is to provide a basic text for new entrants to the field; to act as a resources guide for those who are inexperienced in OH practice; and to discuss contemporary OH issues with those more experienced in the field. It also aims to provide a practical handbook, rather than a theoretical tome.

It is written by relevant experts in the field, all of whom are members of the Association of Occupational Health Nurse Practitioners (UK) and who take an active role either on the board, or as specialist advisers to the board.

Greta Thornbory

Acknowledgements

I would like to express my thanks to the following people for their invaluable contributions to this book.

Firstly to my colleagues in the Association of Occupational Health Nurse Practitioners UK who have contributed by writing the chapters and ensuring their relevance to today's occupational health nursing practice.

To Grace McInnes and James Watson at Routledge for believing we could produce this book and for their advice and support with the project. To Victoria Edwards who came up with an excellent case study. Without these people the book would not have happened.

Thanks must also go to Professor Diana Kloss for writing the foreword, and to Anne Harris and Joan Lewis for their unstinting support on my writing projects. Finally, great thanks to Claire White who reads my scripts and produces an index.

The editor and publisher gratefully acknowledge the permission granted to reproduce the copyright material in this book. Every reasonable effort has been made to trace copyright ownership and to obtain permission for reproduction, and the publisher would be grateful if notified of any corrections that should be incorporated in future reprints or editions of this book.

Greta Thornbory

1 An introduction to occupational health nursing

Greta Thornbory

Learning objectives

After reading this chapter you will be able to:

- discuss the historical aspects of occupational health (OH) nursing
- appreciate the international and national influences on OH and the health and wellbeing of the workers
- describe the role of statutory bodies and the statutory and mandatory aspects of OH nursing registration
- identify the legal and ethical aspects of OH nursing practice
- identify how education and continuing professional development contribute to improving quality of practice.

According to the International Council of Nurses (ICN):[1]

> Nursing encompasses autonomous and collaborative care of individuals of all ages, families, groups and communities, sick or well and in all settings. Nursing includes the promotion of health, prevention of illness, and the care of ill, disabled and dying people. Advocacy, promotion of a safe environment, research, participation in shaping health policy and in patient and health systems management, and education are also key nursing roles.

OH nursing is the branch of nursing that focuses on the care of the working community and certainly fulfils most of the criteria from the ICN definition. The main purpose of this book is to act as a guide and resource for OH nurse practitioners, particularly those new to OH.

OH is not a new medical or health discipline, despite the fact that it is often confused with occupational therapy. Occupational therapy is a holistic healthcare profession that aims to promote health by enabling individuals to perform meaningful and purposeful activities across their lifespan; it deals with ensuring that people can cope with the day-to-day activities of living after accident or illness whilst OH deals specifically with the health and wellbeing of the working population in their place of work. OH aims to work with other disciplines to ensure that the working-age population have the best opportunity to benefit from employment and that they are not injured or made ill by the work they undertake. In the UK people are able to leave school from the age of 16 (soon to rise to 18) and therefore may work from then until retirement. Today, under the Equality Act,[2] as there is no default retirement age people may continue to work for as long as they want. This means that a person's working life may be for over 50 years. We must not forget that in the UK children and young people are allowed to undertake certain work roles after school or college and at weekends, although there are strict laws and guidelines for this. Also there is a large population of unpaid voluntary workers in many organisations, particularly the service sector, who are entitled to the same care as those in paid work.

People spend roughly one-third of their time at work, one-third of their time sleeping and one-third is left for all other activities, such as eating, household and personal chores and socialising. Therefore work is the single activity which dominates the waking hours, so health and wellbeing are important aspects of working life.

The historical aspects of OH and OH nursing

In 1863 Florence Nightingale said 'the hospital should do the sick no harm'[3] and we can apply her sentiments to the workplace by saying 'the work should do the worker no harm'. It has been seen in historical papers and pictures that workers' health has been a source of concern, even as early as ancient Egypt where there are hieroglyphic pictures depicting slaves covering their faces to protect them from the dust created when building the pyramids.

The person regarded as the 'father of occupational medicine' is the seventeenth-century Italian Professor of Medicine, Bernardino Ramazzini. He published in Latin *De Morbis Artificum Diatriba* or *Diseases of Tradesmen and Craftsmen*. This was an exhaustive work outlining the health hazards of chemicals, dust, metals, repetitive or violent motions, odd postures and other disease-causative agents encountered by workers in 52 occupations; these included stone cutters, millers, masons, bricklayers, chemists, metal diggers, potters and glass makers, surgeons and wet nurses as well as learned men. The latter were affected by the more commonly known 'writer's cramp', or as it is known today, repetitive strain injury or work-related upper-limb disorder. Through personal example, Ramazzini demonstrated the importance of talking directly with workers and of visiting workplaces to investigate the working environment in order to improve it. He focused on the need for providing workers with adequate information about health hazards and he suggested practical measures to protect workers from illness and injury.[4]

It was the Industrial Revolution that took place from 1750 to 1850 in the UK that brought about many changes to the working environment. The mechanisation of agriculture, manufacturing, mining and transportation and the advent of technology had a profound effect on the social, economic and cultural conditions in the UK as workers migrated from cottage industries in the country to the factories and mills of the towns and cities. At this time a few philanthropic employers introduced some form of healthcare for their workers – companies whose names are still known today, such as Debenhams, Cadbury, Clarks (shoes) and Coleman's Mustard. Most of this early history of OH, or, as it was known then, industrial health can be read about in Irene Charley's book *The Birth of Industrial Nursing,* published in 1954.[5] As Radwanski[6] wrote in 1978 when the book was reissued, 'OH practitioners . . . should read this account of the courageous efforts to establish OH nursing on a sound professional basis'.

Charley gives details of the first recorded 'occupational health nurse' as Phillipa Flowerday. Miss Flowerday, aged 32, was appointed on 28 October 1878 to Coleman's Mustard in Norwich where she worked with the doctor at the factory in the morning and visited the workers' families in their homes in the afternoons.

Since those early times the working environment has changed a great deal with scientific advances and the advent of electronic and computerised technology. Some of the industrial diseases remain and new ones have taken the place of those that have disappeared. The work of the qualified and registered nurse has changed from that of a handmaiden to the doctor to that of an independent and professionally accountable practitioner governed and guided by his or her own professional body and code of practice.[7]

OH was originally called 'industrial' medicine and nursing because of the Industrial Revolution in the eighteenth century when factory work was so very dangerous, affecting the health and welfare of many people. This was not just adults but also children; they were often given the most dangerous jobs that only small people could do. In those days, and until the later part of the twentieth century, OH was used as a casualty department which treated workers' injuries and illnesses and was more generally called the Medical Department. By the end of the century treatment services had been discontinued by most OH services, with the exception of specific industries such as oil rigs and large construction sites, e.g. the building of the Olympic village in east London. In the UK first aid at work for accidents and injury has been encouraged in light of the First Aid Regulations[8] and easier access to NHS primary care and general practitioners (GPs) in local health centres has encouraged better use of these facilities for minor illness.

The international perspective of OH

In the middle of the twentieth century it was recorded that nearly 2,000 people died from accidents at work per annum in the UK[9] – bearing in mind that few records or statistics were kept on such matters in those days, the figures were probably much higher. By the beginning of the twenty-first century, following the advent of European directives from the EU and much health and safety legislation and guidance, the figure in the UK had reduced to 241 people killed at work per annum.

During this time the name was changed from 'industrial medicine' to 'occupational health' and in 1950 the Joint International Labour Organization (ILO) / World Health

Organization (WHO) issued the first definition of OH, which was updated in 1995 to these three objectives:

1. the maintenance and promotion of workers' health and working capacity
2. the improvement of working environment and work to become conducive to health and safety
3. the development of work organisation and working cultures in a direction which supports health and safety at work and in doing so promotes a positive social climate and smooth operation and may enhance the productivity of the undertaking.

(Twelfth Session of the Joint ILO/WHO
Committee on Occupational Health 1995)

In 2002 the WHO Regional Office for Europe[10] produced guidance for OH professionals and outlined the 11 key functions of an OH service (Figure 1.1).

These key functions relate to OH throughout the EU. Each country interprets these functions according to the political, cultural and social needs of the population and these differences must be respected. Even so, less than 10 per cent of the EU working population has access to OH services.[11]

To address this issue from an OH nursing perspective there is an organisation, the Federation of Occupational Health Nurses within the European Union, which aims to

---

1. Identification and assessment of the health risk in the workplace

2. Surveillance of work environment factors and work practices that affect workers' health, including sanitary installations, canteens and housing, when such facilities are provided by the employer

3. Participation in the development of programmes for the improvement of working practices, as well as testing and evaluating health aspects of new equipment

4. Advice on planning and organisation of work, design of workplaces, choice and maintenance of machinery, equipment and substances used at work

5. Advice on occupational health, safety and hygiene, and on ergonomics and individual and collective protective equipment

6. Surveillance of workers' health in relation to work

7. Promoting the adaptation of work to the worker

8. Collaboration in providing information, training and education in the fields of occupational health, hygiene and ergonomics

9. Contribution to measures of vocational rehabilitation

10. Organisation of first aid and emergency treatment

11. Participation in the analysis of occupational accidents and occupational diseases.

Figure 1.1 Functions of an occupational health service

Source: Alli BO (2008) *Fundamental Principles of Occupational Safety and Health*, 2nd edn. Geneva: International Labour Office.

work together to promote good OH nursing practice throughout the region.[12] There is also a diverse team of OH professionals who undertake this work as it is not just doctors and nurses involved in delivering these 11 functions.[13]

In the UK OH nursing is recognised as a specialist field of nursing, having first been identified as such in 1934, when an industrial nursing course commenced at the (Royal) College of Nursing. Today OH nurses take their place in both the professional OH team and also the public health nursing team. Public health nursing includes health visitors, school nurses, infection control nurses and sexual health nurses, all of whom care for different communities: health visitors for families and under-5s, school nurses for the school-age community, whilst infection control nurses and sexual health nurses deal with specific aspects of care in the community. As OH is a branch of public health this will be explored in depth in Chapter 2.

OH in the twenty-first century

OH nurses care for the working community in their workplace. They must be aware of the hazards and risks to health of all types of employment both in the UK and overseas as many companies have employees working as expats in both Western and developing countries. The promotion of health, prevention of illness and promotion of a safe environment are key to all OH work and will be explored and expanded in Chapters 4, 5 and 7.

It has to be remembered that businesses are there for a specific function – to offer a service or manufacture an item. The health and welfare of the employee have not always been considered a high priority, although there is much evidence to demonstrate that 'good health means good business'. The World Economic Forum in January 2010 reported that its survey, based on over 28,000 employees in 15 countries, found that businesses that took a strategic approach to wellness and engagement were more innovative, more able to retain their staff and more productive overall.[14] Another piece of research from Ipsos MORI[15] showed that FTSE 100 companies that consider the wellness and wellbeing of their employees outperformed the rest of the FTSE 100 by 10 per cent in 2009. On 25 September 2012, BITC Workwell launched a pilot, *Public Reporting on Employee Wellness and Engagement*,[16] that will benchmark all FTSE 100 companies on their reporting of wellness and engagement of their employees to drive business performance in the UK and internationally.

If good health is good business, is it any good for the workers themselves? Yes, say Waddell and Burton,[17] whose report in 2006 reviewed and collated evidence on the question. Their main findings were that:

- Employment is generally the most important means of obtaining adequate economic resources.
- Work meets important psychological needs.
- Work is central to individual identity, social roles and social status.

Conversely, there was a strong association between unemployment and poor mental and physical health and higher mortality. Interestingly, Waddell and Burton also highlighted that work for sick and disabled people should be encouraged where their health permits. Amongst other things their findings were that work:

- is therapeutic
- helps promote recovery and rehabilitation
- leads to better health outcomes
- reduces the risk of long-term incapacity
- reduces poverty
- improves quality of life and wellbeing.

In 2007 and following on from the work of Waddell and Burton, the Secretaries of State for Health and for Work and Pensions commissioned the National Director for Health and Work, Dame Carol Black, to undertake the first ever review of the health of Britain's working-age population. Full details of all the reports and ongoing work can be found at the department's website: http://www.dwp.gov.uk/health-work-and-well-being/about-us. When calling for evidence for her review, Black posed eight main questions:

1. How can we keep working-age people healthy and how can the workplace promote health?
2. How can people best be helped to remain in or quickly return to work when they develop health conditions, including chronic disease or disabilities?
3. How does the age of the person affect the support that is needed?
4. How can we encourage action to improve employee health?
5. What underlies the apparent growth in mental health problems in the working-age population and how can this be addressed?
6. What constitutes effective OH provision and how can it be made available to all?
7. What could be the impact on poverty and social inclusion of a healthier working-age population?
8. What are the costs of working-age ill health to business and what are the benefits to companies of investing in the health of their staff?

The answers to these questions can be found in Black's final report[18] and the government response was published in November 2008.[19] It identified seven key indicators and over 20 subindicators to develop baselines for and measure progress against. The seven key indicators are:

1. knowledge and perceptions about the importance of work to health and health to work
2. improving the promotion of health and wellbeing at work
3. reducing the incidence of work-related ill health and injuries and their causes
4. reducing the proportion of people out of work due to ill health
5. improving the self-reported health status of the working-age population
6. the experience of working-age people in accessing appropriate and timely health service support
7. improving business productivity and performance.

Since that time a number of recommendations have been implemented. A Council for Work & Health has been set up and details of the work of this council can be found on their website at http://www.councilforworkandhealth.org.uk, where it says that:

> OH services are delivered collaboratively by a wide range of professional groups. Each one contributes its own particular blend of skills and competencies, some of which are unique, and some of which are shared with other professions.
>
> The Council for Work & Health brings together the professional bodies which represent these groups to provide an authoritative and representative 'single voice' on health and well-being issues. It also provides an opportunity for co-ordinated and integrated working on all issues which impact on health and well-being services and facilitates information sharing to promote improvement.

OH nursing is represented on the council by the Association of Occupational Health Nurse Practitioners (AOHNP) and it takes a very active part.

Whilst people at work are deemed to be 'fit for work', many of them work with chronic medical conditions, both physical and mental, as well as all manner of disabilities. The knowledge and skills required by OH nurses when advising employers and employees on an individual's fitness to work, the reasonable adjustments they will need and rehabilitation following a period of absence will be covered in depth in Chapter 6. In today's economic climate the OH nurse's role is key to case management when dealing with absence from work. Following the Black report work has been ongoing on sickness absence, absence management and rehabilitation after accident, injury and/or illness and this will be explored in depth in Chapters 6 and 7.

Since the publication of the report in 2008 and the then government response there has been a change of government. For the most up-to-date political position it is necessary to keep an eye on the Health, Work and Well-being website. The last publication appears to be the baseline indicators report[20] published just after the change of government in December 2010. The issues of public health will be addressed in depth in Chapter 2.

Although evidence-based practice will be woven throughout this book, Chapter 9 is devoted to developing an understanding of epidemiology and its place in OH so that all care is evidence-based. The final chapter will cover that all-important aspect of quality assurance and auditing practice, a factor that the Black report highlighted as necessary for all OH services.

OH nursing today

OH nurses are regarded as specialist nurses by the nursing and midwifery regulator, the Nursing and Midwifery Council (NMC). The NMC exists to safeguard the health and wellbeing of the public and was established under the Nursing and Midwifery Order 2001 ('the order') and came into being on 1 April 2002. It replaced the previous council as there were significant changes under the new Act.

The role of the NMC is to set standards of education, training, conduct and performance so that nurses and midwives can deliver high-quality healthcare consistently throughout their careers. It also ensures that nurses and midwives keep their skills and knowledge up to date and uphold professional standards. They have clear and transparent processes to investigate nurses and midwives who fall short of our standards. To practise lawfully as a registered nurse in the UK, the practitioner must hold a current and valid registration with the NMC. The title 'registered nurse' can only be granted to those holding such registration. This protected title is laid down in the Nurses, Midwives and Health Visitors Act 1997 and is repeated as an offence in the 2001 legislation.

It is therefore necessary in the UK for anyone working as (and calling him- or herself) an OH nurse to hold a current and valid registration. However, even though OH nursing is regarded as specialist area of practice there is no legal requirement for employers to employ specialist practitioner nurses, i.e. nurses who have undergone additional specialist education and training. This area is quite complex to explain.

The NMC lays down *Standards of Proficiency for Specialist Community Public Health Nurses*[21] which are then interpreted by the relevant educating body, usually a university. Once an educating body, usually a university, has designed a suitable course it is then validated by the NMC. Some universities prefer to offer non-NMC-validated courses for nurses working in OH. As there is no legal requirement for employers to employ nurses registered with the NMC as specialist practitioners, this is no problem providing the registered nurse fulfils the requirements of his/her professional code of practice, which states: 'As a professional you are personally accountable for actions and omissions in your practice, and must always be able to justify your decisions.'[7] Later in the same code it states that nurses must recognise and work within their limits of competence and as OH is a specialist area of practice there is a limit to the knowledge, skills and understanding of a nurse who has not undertaken specialist education and training in this field.

There has been much criticism of the NMC-validated courses; indeed, the Council for Work and Health has prepared a report[22] and held talks with the NMC on this topic based on the findings of a review of the situation undertaken by Kirk.[23] Her findings were that the current specialist training structures have a number of weaknesses:

1. There is no requirement for university teaching staff on the courses where OH students are taught to be OH-qualified, or even to have OH experience.
2. There is financial pressure to fill student places so the course is kept generic in order to accept as many students as possible, therefore diluting the OH content.
3. There are relatively small numbers of OH nurse students and a tendency to cater for the majority, i.e. health visitors.
4. There is no detailed curriculum for specific public health genres, such as OH, defined by the NMC.
5. There is a perceived bureaucracy amongst experienced nurses: OH nurses don't immediately appreciate why they can't teach on a specialist programme if they only have a certificate (OHNC) or diploma (OHND) because degree courses weren't available when they trained.

These factors are compounded by nurses not being able to access courses because of financial problems and even if they do have funding they may not be able to access the

NMC requirements of a 'practice teacher' for similar reasons, given in point 5 above. Even those OH nurses with specialist qualifications at degree or master's level are precluded from being a practice teacher if they do not have an NMC-recognised teaching qualification, and their acceptance of teaching qualifications is quite narrow. Lastly, employers are not happy to spend money on training their OH nurses to teach; they pay them to provide OH services to their employees!

At the time of writing the NMC education role is under review and it is worth checking the NMC and the Council for Work and Health websites for up-to-date information.

The specialist practitioner standards of proficiency outlined[21] by the NMC are:

- surveillance and assessment of the population
- collaborative working
- working with, and for, communities
- developing health programmes and services and reducing inequalities
- policy and strategy development and implementation
- research and development
- promoting and protecting the population
- developing quality and risk management within an evaluative culture
- strategic leadership
- ethically managing self, people and resources.

Bearing in mind these proficiencies are related to all public health nurses, including health visitors and school nurses, whose populations are vastly different from OH nurses, are they still relevant for today's OH practice? Kirk[23] argues that these standards were relevant in the past with the industrial nurse but not so relevant with the case management and rehabilitation role of the OH nurse in the twenty-first century. One can counterargue that the terms are broad and open to interpretation. For example, collaborative working, working for communities, developing health programmes and reducing inequalities all encompass the case management and rehabilitation role. It indicates that there is a clear need for experienced and well-qualified OH nurses to be involved with the development of curriculum and syllabus for OH nurse education and training. Preferably this would be in a multidisciplinary setting with other professional disciplines who are part of the OH team rather than with health visitors and school nurses who do not deal with the working population on a regular basis.

If these NMC standards of proficiency are to be interpreted correctly to prepare nurses for their work in OH then it is necessary to consider what they are required to do to fulfil the 11 functions of an OH service.[10] The functions of any OH service will depend entirely on the type of company/organisation and the work it does. These can be divided roughly into public bodies, such as the NHS and local government etc. or private companies from international organisations employing many thousands of people, manufacturing or service industries and SMEs and charities.

SME is the collective term for small and medium-size enterprises, the definition of which is laid down by the European Commission.[24] Put simply, any organisation with fewer than 250 employees but more than 50 is medium, those with fewer than 50 but more than 10 are small and fewer than 10 are regarded as micro. This is particularly important to consider because in the UK 99.9 per cent of employers employing 49 per cent of the workforce fall into the SME brackets. Because of the small number of employees these organisations are less likely to employ or have access to OH services.[25] To address this issue the Black report recommended that an advice service should be made available and now a 'health for work advice line' is available to SMEs in the UK – see http://www.dwp.gov.uk/health-work-and-well-being/our-work/oh-adviceline. Today there are many OH service providers to SMEs and the Faculty of Occupational Medicine has developed a system for assessing that they are 'safe effective quality occupational health services'.[26] The work of SMEs and other OH services will be explored in depth in Chapter 8 whilst quality assurance and audit will be explored in Chapter 10.

In 2001 Baranski and Whitaker[27] produced a document describing the role of the OH nurse in workplace health management. The European contributors to this EU paper included three experienced and well-qualified OH nurses from the UK. They have determined that OH nurses may fulfil several often interrelated and complementary roles as:

- clinician
- specialist
- manager
- coordinator
- adviser
- health educator
- counsellor
- researcher.

As noted, these roles are interrelated and it is difficult to explore each one individually, but suffice it to say that throughout this book these roles will be explored within the dimensions of the different chapter topics.

In 2005 the At Work Partnership published their research report on the *Performance Indicators and Benchmarking in OH Nursing.*[28] This research was undertaken on 473 OH nurses who came from all sectors of employment, some working across more than one sector. It is not known exactly how many OH nurses are practising in the UK; a rough estimate by Kirk[23] is that between 5 and 7,000 are practising, 4,500 of whom are qualified in OH. So this cannot really be taken as a truly representative sample but it is the best there is to date. One of the findings of the At Work report (Figure 1.2) demonstrates what the respondents thought were the essential OH nursing functions and reflected the different types of OH practised in particular organisations, e.g. travel health, and advice would only be needed for the companies with employees travelling abroad on business as it is not the role of the OH to duplicate the work of the GP, whereas specific immunisations would be required in certain industries and the NHS as part of health surveillance and the protection of the worker. Again all these functions are addressed in depth in subsequent chapters of this book.

1 Confidential handling of health and personal data (95%)	2 Assessment of fitness for work (88%)	3 Delivering health surveillance (84%)	4 Interpretation of health surveillance (84%)
5 Disability assessments and adjustments (81%)	6 Assessing risks to mental health (81%)	7 Analysing of pre-employment/ preplacement questionnaires (77%)	8 Interpreting and advising on OH law (76%)
9 Developing fitness-for-work standards (71%)	10 Confidential counselling (68%)	11 Health and safety risk assessment (66%)	12 Sharps/needlestick prevention and management (63%)
13 Display screen equipment assessments (62%)	14 Vocational rehabilitation (61%)	15 Advising on work organisation and design (59%)	16 Delivering return-to-work interviews (58%)
17 Monitoring work-related accident, injury and illness data (58%)	18 Attendance monitoring (53%)	19 Provision of training and education (53%)	20 Immunisation (50%)
21 Cost–benefit analysis of OH interventions (50%)	22 Organisation of first aid and first-aid training (44%)	23 Provision of personal protective equipment (44%)	24 General health and wellness screening (39%)
25 Travel health advice/provision (25%)	26 Home/off-site visits to workers on sick leave (23%)		

Figure 1.2 Essential occupational health (OH) nursing functions

Note: the figures show the percentages of OH nurses who rate each function as essential. Courtesy of the At Work Partnership.

Confidentiality

It is interesting to note that singularly the most important essential function for 95 per cent of respondents was the confidential handling of health and personal data. Confidentiality is probably the one aspect of OH that nurses find difficulty in dealing with when they are frequently asked to divulge information about employees' health, medical condition or diagnosis by the human resources (HR) department or line manager. This causes OH nurses considerable stress and the answers are not simple. There are a number of legal and ethical factors to be considered.

The legal aspects

The Data Protection Act 1998
The Data Protection Act 1998, Employment Practices Code[29] states that workers have a legitimate expectation that they can keep their personal health information private and that the employer will respect that privacy. It goes on to state that

interpretation of medical information should be left to suitably qualified health professionals. Information about workers' health is regarded as 'sensitive data' in the code and employers must only collect that data which is necessary for health and safety reasons, to prevent discrimination, to satisfy legal requirements or if the worker has given explicit consent. It goes on to state that employers should not compromise the communications between workers and health professionals in an OH service. OH nurses should all be aware of this code and download a copy for easy reference.

Human Rights Act

Lewis and Thornbory[30] state that confidentiality in the workplace has a human rights perspective with the right to a private and family life. Therefore it reiterates the Data Protection Act code in that health information on employees should only be gathered if necessary for the reasons given in the code and used appropriately and treated confidentially.

Access to Medical Reports Act 1988

This act gives individuals the right of access to any medical report relating to them supplied by a doctor for employment or insurance purposes. On its terms it applies only to reports requested from a registered medical practitioner who has been responsible for clinical care. It therefore does not strictly speaking apply to reports from nurses or other health professionals or to most OH reports. However, good OH practice today dictates that in order to be able to give informed consent employees should know what is to be said about them before a report is made to management, and this has been strengthened by advice from the General Medical Council on confidentiality.[29,31,32]

Professional aspects

OH nurses are governed by their professional registering body, the NMC, by their code of practice[7] and additional advice on confidentiality.[32,33] This of course relates to all nurses in all settings, not just OH. The key clauses in both documents are:

- You must respect people's rights to confidentiality.
- You must ensure people are informed about how and why information is shared by those who will be providing care.
- You must disclose information if you believe someone may be at risk of harm, in line with the laws of the country in which you are practising.

These all apply to OH practice and in particular the last clause. This may be necessary with people at work whose health may put themselves or others at risk. Of course it is always advisable to get the person's consent, and good practice is always to ask patients/clients to consent to disclosure as this prevents any difficult situations at a later date. Lewis and Thornbory[30] provides a number of templates which can be downloaded and adapted for use by OH practitioners, which include a management referral form where the employee can give consent to a report being prepared by OH, employee consent to disclosure form and a medical report consent form.

Other guidance on confidentiality in OH can be found in Kloss and Ballard,[34] the guidance on ethics for occupational physicians[35] and guidance on confidentiality available to AOHNP members on their website. More information about confidentiality and consent is dealt with in the relevant places throughout the book.

Competence

Earlier in this chapter the NMC Code of Practice was quoted as saying that nurses must recognise and work within their limits of competence, but what exactly is meant by competence? It is a term that is also used in health and safety codes of practice so it is particularly relevant to OH nurses.

If one considers what 'competence' actually means, then usually one can think of two or three words to describe it. If you look at dictionary definitions of competence the words that one usually finds are 'skilled', 'knowledgeable', 'expertise', along with able, capable and well-qualified and competence is also defined by behaviour. A useful way of remembering what competence means is the equation $C = KSU$, where competence equals knowledge, skills and understanding. Here is an example.

In OH practice OH nurses may have to deal with overseas business travellers and this may involve the administration of immunisations. In other areas of practice the nurse will be *au fait* with giving injections as prescribed by a doctor but in OH such practice is undertaken under a local protocol with a Patient Group Direction (PGD).[36] The OH nurse will need to have the following evidence-based knowledge and skills on overseas travel and the administration of immunisations to undertake this work:

- How long before travel will immunisations need to be given to protect the worker and what time needs to be allowed between doses and/or different types of immunisations to complete the course?
- The type of immunisations, their contraindications and side-effects
- How and where it is administered
- How to deal with anaphylaxis and be up to date with procedures
- How to dispose of clinical waste in a community setting, i.e. outside a healthcare facility
- What other information is needed for travellers to specific countries and where to go for that up-to-date information.

This list is not exhaustive but gives an indication of the knowledge, skills and understanding required to be competent in one aspect of OH practice. This is known as the knowledge 'that' – the theory that underpins the practice, rather than the knowledge 'how', which is the skill required to administer the immunisation. Rogers[37] explains

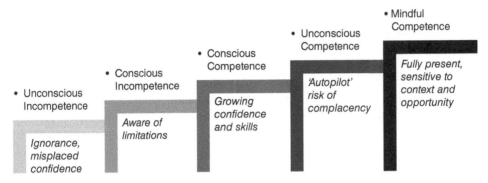

Figure 1.3 Ladder of competence

the different aspects of competence using the 'ladder of competence' (Figure 1.3). The two most dangerous levels are 1 and 5, the former where we don't know what we don't know and the latter where we think we know it all!

Gaining knowledge, skills and experience in OH practice will help to develop the nurse from a 'novice to expert'; although not specifically on OH practice we can read more about this concept in Benner's book.[38] The Royal College of Nursing guidance on OH nursing career and competence development, which is based on the NHS Knowledge and Skills Framework, has developed OH nurse competence dimensions and level descriptors for practice[39] from competent through experience to expert under the following headings:

- self-assessment
- core transferable skills
- core leadership and management skills
- core quality assurance and research skills
- legal and ethical issues
- risk assessment
- public health, health promotion, protection and surveillance
- psychological and psychosocial interventions
- attendance management, case management and rehabilitation
- ergonomics
- occupational hygiene
- maintaining safety and accident control.

These headings coincide very well with the chapters in this book and, where they overlap, such as legal and ethical issues, transferable skills and self-assessment, these will be woven thought the book.

Competence can only be gained through education, training and experience, where the education is gained from attending a specialist OH course which builds on a first-level nursing course and subsequent refresher courses, where on-the-job, practical training is given and experience gained under OH nurse supervision at a practical work placement. As independent practitioners accountable for their own actions, OH nurses have to determine for themselves whether or not they are competent to do the job and take on the responsibility. This clearly demonstrates the need for continuing professional development (CPD) once a specialist qualification is obtained.

Continuing professional development

With annual re-registering, the NMC requires that all nurses sign on their own cognisance that they have undertaken CPD and kept up to date to a minimum of 35 hours of learning activity in the previous 3 years.[40] The NMC recommends that CPD may take a number of forms, including:

- e-learning
- journals
- specialist forums
- individual study
- work-based learning
- formal CPD study days.

The learning activity must be what suits individual practitioners' own learning styles and meets individual need. It should identify core learning needs and those that are specialist to the field of practice. This is often achieved with the help of professional (clinical) supervision[41] or annual job performance reviews. Once you have undertaken the learning activity the NMC asks you to keep a record of that activity and suggests you should reflect on and record the learning activity related to the work under the following headings:

- the nature of the learning activity – what you did
- a description of the learning activity and what it consisted of
- the outcome of the learning activity – how the learning related to your work
- you should also note any influence on or changes to your practice and any follow-up learning needed.

OH nurses who work outside the healthcare setting and find that employers are not helpful with this aspect of professional practice may find it useful to note that the NMC has a section for employers,[42] where it includes HR managers, and outlines the employer's responsibilities and gives guidance when employing nurses.

Conclusion

OH nursing is a vital nursing specialism caring for a vast population of (potentially) healthy working people. It is vital to the economy of the country in keeping employees at work, preventing them from ill health and accident, whether caused by work or not, and is vital in helping to support the family economy. Waddell and Burton's[17] work demonstrated that work is good for health and wellbeing and that unemployment is positively detrimental. For OH nurses to undertake this specialist role they have to follow international and national professional guidelines. This chapter has considered the historical, international and national perspectives of OH and OH nursing and the practice that is required in the twenty-first century in the UK today. It has considered the ongoing work and research in this specialism at a national and professional level as well as the legal and professional aspects of confidentiality and competence in the role of the OH nurse. It is not possible to cover every aspect of this vast topic in one chapter but the references and web links should lead you to further and indepth reading of this subject. The important and actual day-to-day work of the OH nurse will be visited in each of the subsequent chapters, with this one acting as a basis to guide professional practice.

References

1 International Council of Nursing (12.04.2010) *Nursing Definition*. Available online at: http://www.icn.ch/about-icn/icn-definition-of-nursing (accessed 16.10.12).
2 Equality Act 2010.
3 Nightingale F (1863) *Notes on Hospitals,* 3rd edn. Preface.
4 http://www.collegiumramazzini.org/about03.asp.
5 Charley I H (1954) *The Birth of Industrial Nursing.* London: Baillière, Tindall and Cox.
6 Radwanski D (1978) The birth of industrial nursing. *Br J Ind Med* 35 (4): 339.
7 Nursing and Midwifery Council (2008) *The Code: Standards of conduct, performance and ethics for nurses and midwives.* London: NMC.
8 Health and Safety (First Aid) Regulations 1981 SI No. 917.
9 Gifford P (2008) From phenol poisoning to stress: 60 years of health and safety. *Health Care Risk Rep* 14 (8) 18–19.
10 Lie A, Baranski B, Husman K, Westerholm P (2002) *Good Practice in Occupational Health Services: A contribution to workplace health.* Europe: WHO Regional Office. Available online at: http://www.euro.who.int/__data/assets/pdf_file/0007/115486/E77650.pdf (accessed 10.01.13).
11 http://www.euro.who.int/en/what-we-do/health-topics/environment-and-health/occupational-health (accessed 10.01.13).
12 http://www.fohneu.org.
13 Thornbory G (2009) *Public Health Nursing.* Oxford: Wiley Blackwell, pp. 158–162.
14 Dornan A (2010) *The Wellness Imperative: Creating more effective organisations.* Report to the World Economic Forum. Geneva: Right Management. Available online at: http://www3.weforum.org/docs/WEF_HE_WellnessImperativeCreatingMoreEffective Organizations_Report_2010.pdf.
15 BITC/Ipsos MORI (2010) *FTSE 100 Research: Public Reporting Trends.* London: BITC.
16 Business In The Community (2012) http://www.bitc.org.uk/workplace/health_and_well-being/the_workwell_movement/workwell_ftse_100.html.
17 Waddell G, Burton A K (2006) *Is Work Good for Your Health and Well-Being?* Norwich: TSO. http://www.dwp.gov.uk/docs/hwwb-is-work-good-for-you.pdf (accessed 09.01.13).
18 Black C (2008) *Working for a Healthier Tomorrow.* London: TSO. Available online at: http://www.dwp.gov.uk/docs/hwwb-working-for-a-healthier-tomorrow.pdf (accessed 09.01.13).
19 Department of Work and Pensions (2008) *Improving Health and Changing Lives.* DWP: London. Available online at: http://www.dwp.gov.uk/docs/hwwb-improving-health-and-work-changing-lives.pdf.

20 http://www.dwp.gov.uk/docs/hwwb-baseline-indicators.pdf.

21 NMC (2004) *Standards of Proficiency for Specialist Community Public Health Nurses.* London: NMC.

22 Harriss A (2011) *The Challenge of Preparing Nurses Practicing in the Workplace Setting Competent to Promote, Improve and Maintain the Health of the Working Age Population.* London: Council for Work and Health. http://www.councilforworkand health.org.uk/images/uploads/library/Nurse%20training/Final%20Paper%20from%20 Anne%20Harriss%20with%20appendices.pdf (accessed 16.01.13).

23 Kirk H (2009) *Issues in OH Nurse Education: A short review.* London: BITC.

24 European Commission (2005) *The New SME Definition.* Available online at: http:// ec.europa.eu/enterprise/policies/sme/files/sme_definition/sme_user_guide_en.pdf (accessed 17.01.13).

25 http://data.gov.uk/dataset/small_and_medium_sized_enterprise_statistics_sme_for_ the_uk_and_regions (accessed 17.01.13).

26 http://www.fom.ac.uk/standards-for-occupational-health-services/seqohs (accessed 17.01.13).

27 Baranski B, Whitaker S (2001) *The Role of the Occupational Health Nurse in Workplace Health Management.* Bilthoven: WHO European Centre for Environment and Health. http://www.who.int/occupational_health/regions/en/oeheurnursing.pdf (accessed 17.01.13).

28 Ballard J, Silcox S, Suff P (2005) *Performance Indicators and Benchmarking in OH Nursing: A research report.* Barnet: The At Work Partnership. http://www.atwork partnership.co.uk/research/Performance_indicators.pdf (accessed 24.01.13).

29 Information Commissioner (2011) *Employment Practices Code: Part 4: Information about workers health.* London: ICO. http://www.ico.gov.uk/for_organisations/data_pro tection/topic_guides/~/media/documents/library/Data_Protection/Detailed_specialist_ guides/the_employment_practices_code.ashx (accessed 18.02.13).

30 Lewis J, Thornbory G (2010) *Employment Law and Occupational Health: A practical handbook.* Oxford: Wiley-Blackwell.

31 Kloss D (2009) *Consent and Confidentiality in Occupational Health Reports.* http:// www.fom.ac.uk/wp-content/uploads/conffomoct09kloss.pdf (accessed 18.01.13).

32 Kloss D (2010) *Occupational Health Law,* 5th edn. Oxford: Wiley-Blackwell.

33 NMC (2009) *Confidentiality.* London: NMC. Available online at: www.nmc-uk.org (accessed 17.01.13).

34 Kloss D, Ballard J (2012) *Discrimination Law and Occupational Health Practice.* Barnet: The At Work Partnership.

35 Litchfield P, Brecker N (eds) (2012) *Ethics Guidance for Occupational Health Practice.* London: Faculty of Occupational Medicine.

36 NMC (2007) *Standards for Medicines Management.* London: NMC.

37 Rogers J (2007) *Adults Learning,* 5th edn. Berkshire: Open University Press.

38 Benner P (1984) *From Novice to Expert: Excellence and power in clinical nursing practice.* New Jersey: Prentice Hall.

39 RCN (2011) *Occupational Health Nursing: Career and competence development.* London, RCN. Available online at: http://www.rcn.org.uk/__data/assets/pdf_file/0007/481759/ Occ_health_nursing_career_and_competence_development.pdf (accessed 23.01.13).

40 NMC (2011) *The Prep Handbook.* London: NMC. Available online at: http://www. nmc-uk.org/Documents/Standards/NMC_Prep-handbook_2011.pdf (accessed 24.01.13).

41 Elliot R (2010) Education and continuing professional development of public health nurses. In: Thornbory G (ed.) *Public Health Nursing.* Oxford: Wiley Blackwell.

42 NMC (undated) *Employers and Managers.* Available online at: http://www.nmc-uk. org/Employers-and-managers.

Public health

2

Kate Kyne

Learning objectives

After reading this chapter you will be able to:

- discuss the meaning of public health
- appreciate the changes in public health over time
- identify the inequalities in health and discuss ways to reduce these
- discuss the challenges that occupational health (OH) nurses face with the public health agenda.

Introduction

With government policy acknowledging the importance of the public health contribution of all nurses, midwives and health visitors, this chapter highlights the importance of OH nurses focusing on and adapting their working patterns to encompass the public health agenda. OH nurses are in the front line in helping to protect and promote the health and wellbeing of the working population. This chapter will explore the key role that OH nurses play in the public health agenda. It will also cover the most recent Department of Health advice and demonstrate how OH nurses have always been leading the way by partnership working, engagement and encouraging people to participate in decisions about their health which ultimately will have a positive effect on the business.

What is public health?

An early definition of public health is from Winslow. In the 1920s, Winslow stated that public health was:

the science and art of preventing disease, prolonging life, and promoting mental and physical health and efficiency through organised community efforts for the sanitation of the environment, the control of communicable infections, the education of the individual in personal hygiene, the organisation of medical and nursing services for the early diagnosis and preventive treatment of disease, and the development of social machinery to ensure to every individual a standard of living adequate for the maintenance of health, so organising these benefits as to enable every citizen to realise their birthright of health and longevity.[1]

A more recent definition from the Department of Health states:

Public health is about helping people to stay healthy, and protecting them from threats to their health. The government wants everyone to be able to make healthier choices, regardless of their circumstances, and to minimise the risk and impact of illness.[2]

Therefore public health can be seen as the science of protecting and improving the health of communities through education, promotion of healthy lifestyles and research for disease and injury prevention. Public health professionals analyse the effect on health of genetics, personal choice and the environment in order to develop programmes that protect the health of the family and community. Overall, public health is concerned with protecting the health of the entire population. Within the field of OH, the population can be classed as the workforce.

Public health professionals try to prevent problems from happening or recurring by implementing educational programmes, developing policies, administering services and conducting research, in contrast to more generic clinical professionals, such as the doctors and nurses within the NHS settings, who focus primarily on treating individuals after they become sick or injured. It is also a field that is concerned with limiting health disparities and a large part of public health is the fight for healthcare equity, quality and accessibility.

The developing role of public health

People in the twenty-first century expect services to be fast, high-quality, responsive and fitted around their lives. All public services should put the person who uses them at their heart. This applies to health and social care because all care is personal.[3]

The above statement covers the vision for healthcare across the UK and indicates the changes in the way services are delivered since the beginning of the NHS in 1948. The role and contribution of public health are becoming increasingly more important in the prevention of illness and the promotion of wellbeing.

In 2000, the government published the NHS Plan;[4] this 10-year programme was aimed to address the difficulties faced by the NHS and to tackle the issues around patient-centred care. The current focus is on transforming the NHS into a high-quality, high-performance system engaged in a continuous cycle of improvement. This stage of reform is set out in the NHS Next Stage Review publications by Darzi, *High Quality Care for All,*[5] *A High Quality Workforce*[6] and *Our Vision for Primary and Community Care.*[7]

Darzi's vision is structured around four main themes, which can be seen throughout many of the domains set within the Safe Effective Quality Occupational Health Service (SEQOHS) accreditation standards.[8] The aim of these standards is to support the achievement of safe, appropriate and effective quality service by auditing against key standards (discussed more fully in Chapters 8 and 10):

- high-quality care for patients and the public – an NHS that works in partnership to prevent ill health, providing care that is personal, effective and safe
- quality at the heart of everything we do – high-quality care throughout the NHS
- freedom to focus on quality – putting frontline staff in control
- high-quality work in the NHS – supporting staff to deliver high-quality care.

One of the biggest changes within the NHS has been the increased focus on prevention of illness and the maintenance of good health as opposed to cure and the move to provide more care within the community, including the workplace, rather than the acute hospital setting.

Inequalities in health

The UK government has identified the need to tackle the causes and consequences of health inequalities and made a commitment to take action and change this. The core to this is to have an impact on avoidable ill health. The government's aim is to reduce health inequalities by also tackling the wider social factors of health such as poverty, unemployment, poor education, poor housing, and poorer environments and communities.

The conclusions from the 1980 Black report[9] were also repeated in the independent inquiry in 1998 into inequalities in health,[10] chaired by Sir Donald Acheson. These findings show that there were health inequalities in Britain and that poverty had a significant impact on health. The report also states that, although the mortality rates have decreased over the past five decades, unacceptable inequalities persisted. The inquiry also found the root causes of ill health could be traced back to a number of social determinants such as education, lifestyle, income and employment.

The Acheson inquiry appears to have influenced the government's policies to address health inequalities; these include the Green Paper *Our Healthier Nation,*[11] the White Paper *Saving Lives,*[12] *Wellbeing in Wales,*[13] *Improving Health in Scotland,*[14] *A Healthier Future: A twenty year vision for health and wellbeing in Northern Ireland 2005–2025,*[15] *Delivering for Health,*[16] and *Better Health, Better Care.*[17] All of these policies focused on three main areas to bring about the change that would be required:

1. Setting targets: After Acherson's report, and the following government policies, health inequalities became a government priority. With the Public Service Agreement of 2002,[18] the overarching target was to reduce inequalities by 10 per cent by 2010

by measuring infant mortality and life expectancy at birth, with supporting targets to reduce mortality rates for heart disease and stroke and related disease by at least 40 per cent by 2010. Additional aims were to reduce mortality rates from cancers by 20 per cent in people under 75, and reduce adult smoking rates to 21 per cent or less by 2010.

The government followed on with *Tackling Health Inequalities: A programme for action*;[19] this was to show what was required to meet the 2010 national targets on life expectancy and infant mortality. This clearly set out NHS interventions required to help achieve these targets. The plans were more clearly defined in the government paper *Choosing Health*[20] and the delivery plan[21] that followed. It was recognised that action was required both within and outside the NHS and at all levels (national, regional and local) to tackle these health inequalities, and that it would take resources and expertise to be able to ensure that these targets were attained and all actions delivered.

2. Shift to primary care: It has been recognised that primary-based care for many is far more accessible to the general population, and that this more local approach can reduce hospital admissions for many conditions. According to the Department of Health in its White Paper, *Our Health, Our Care, Our Say: A new direction for community services*,[3] they felt that there was a need for a radical and sustained shift in the way services would be delivered to ensure more personalised and accessible health programmes were available to fit with people's busy lives. The paper also suggests that people wanted a seamless health and social care provision to support them to remain healthy or to assist in making life choices to change habits which could be causing ill health. In 2008, Darzi[7] set out how the vision for services should continue to grow and develop over the next 10 years. It could be argued that primary and community care should increasingly continue to play a vital role in assisting people to live healthy lives. This should not just be available from local general practitioners (GPs), community nurses, pharmacists and other community-based health professionals, but also from OH professionals within the workplace.

3. Changing and influencing behaviour: Health is affected by a number of factors, including where we live, our income, genetics, education and our social relationships. The government clearly recognised that there was a two-way approach to this, emphasising that the individual and the government had equal responsibilities. In 2006 the Department of Health stated:

> We each have a responsibility for our own health and wellbeing throughout our lives. At the same time, the government has a role in promoting healthier, longer lives lived to the full. We will build on, and strengthen the opportunities for improving the health of the population first set out in our document *Choosing Health*.[3]

Over the last decade life expectancy and health in general have improved, but the health inequalities remain evident in some areas of disadvantaged groups. The government continued to show commitment in understanding the health inequalities and how to reduce these, and so commissioned a review in 2010 to devise an evidence-based strategy. Marmot[22] amongst others, suggests that the key areas that affect health are still employment, skills, education and standard of living. It can therefore be seen that OH nurses will have an increasingly important and pivotal role in creating the opportunities for people to live healthy lives, prevent ill health, continue to influence public and health policies, and also have a positive effect on their organisation's productivity and financial standing, whether this is in the private or public sector.

Activity

What does wellbeing mean to you? Take 10 minutes to consider this and how you feel it links to the workplace and the benefits to your organisation.

What is wellbeing?

Definitions of wellbeing generally relate to people's experience of their quality of life. As defined by Waddell and Burton,[23] 'The subjective state of being healthy, happy, contented, comfortable and satisfied with one's quality of life. It includes physical, material, social, emotional ("happiness"), and development and activity dimensions.'

As a large proportion of adults' time is spent within the workplace, employers should play an important role in assisting their employees to achieve a good quality of life. The workplace, in particular the OH team or individual, should also be seen to encourage employees to improve their health.

The Chartered Institute of Personnel and Development (CIPD) looks more at individuals and their wellbeing having an impact on the organisation, and so uses the following definition of wellbeing, which balances the needs of the employee with those of the organisation:[24] 'creating an environment to promote a state of contentment which allows an employee to flourish and achieve their full potential for the benefit of themselves and their organisation'. This can be seen to be linked to employee engagement and so create an environment that people will want to work within, with a feeling of being valued and supported.

The government's strategy paper, *Health, Work and Wellbeing – Caring for our future*[25] was clearly focused on developing and delivering strategies for preventing ill health and supporting those with health conditions to remain within the work environment and reducing absence rates due to health issues and incapacity for work.

Dame Carol Black very clearly suggests that the importance of employees and their value to the workplace is key, and this is supported by the Institute of Directors in 2006:

> A business's most valuable asset is, and will always be, the dedicated staff that devote themselves to delivering the work of the organisation. Healthy and fit staff are essential to ensuring a company remains efficient and profitable. None of us doubt that good staff management practices ensure that our workforce delivers

our aims, but many of us forget that unless we help them manage their health, fitness and wellbeing, many of our workers can and will fall ill. Surveys of our workers show that they value these aspects of their work more than just financial rewards. People want to perform to the best of their ability.

We know that work is good for people. It provides economic stability as well as being a valuable source of social interaction both for the individual and the community within which they work. Fit, healthy employees deliver profitable businesses which in turn allow the UK to remain one of the most prosperous and best places to work and live.[26]

The role of occupational health nurses in the public health agenda

For far too long it has been assumed that people with health conditions should be protected from work; however, as the evidence has already shown, this is clearly detrimental to an individual's health and wellbeing, as work, employment, standards of living and social relationships all have a direct impact on health.

There are still around 300,000 people a year falling out of work and into the welfare system because of health-related issues and conditions. A significant number of these cases could well be prevented with the appropriate support being provided by a competent OH professional.

The UK spends around £13 million a year on health-related benefits, with employers facing a cost of around £9 million for occupational sick pay and other associated costs.[27] On top of the financial cost, there are social effects: once out of work, an individual's health is more likely to deteriorate and there is a higher risk of falling into poverty, which can also have a very detrimental effect not only on individuals, but also on the family and the community in which they live.

In their review, Black and Frost[27] suggest the establishment of a health and work assessment and advisory service to make OH advice more readily available to both employers and employees, thereby improving sickness absence management.

With the launch of the Public Health Responsibility Deal in England in March 2011,[28] there was a key aim to reduce sickness absence. It is relevant to employers and employees in all sectors of the economy, and was designed to provide the relevant tools and structure to enable employers to look at and address the main public health issues facing their employees. With 175 partners from private, public and voluntary sectors signed up, they pledged to record and work towards reducing sickness absence. Members were also committed to supporting their employees to lead a healthier lifestyle. This responsibility, especially within the NHS, was passed to the OH team, as they were seen to be the leaders on promoting and supporting public health programmes, which in turn, supports the organisation's policies in reducing sickness absence.

Many employers recognise the benefits and importance of the OH role in supporting reduction in sickness absence, and report that absence is a barrier to productivity. It has been shown that, indeed, 90 per cent of employers agree they have a responsibility to encourage employees to be physically and mentally active.[29]

It has been recognised that GPs also play a key role in supporting people back into the work environment, and the Department for Work and Pensions (2013)[30] makes recommendations to revise the fit note guidance and do more to improve GPs' knowledge and awareness of the benefit system and evidence on health and work, in particular their understanding of mental health and employment.

It is also recognised that the workforce is ageing and that this will have an effect on all workplaces across the country. The needs of older workers must be taken into consideration and appropriate support and health programmes put in place to ensure people are able to continue working to a later age. It can also be argued that as much support and OH care needs to be focused on younger workers as they commence employment, to ensure the right services are available to support them and to improve their resilience for their working life.

Addressing the needs of employees who have mental health problems has also been an area that has needed focus, and with the introduction of the Equality Act in 2010, employers are more aware of their duties, especially under the sections related to disability. The act defines a disability. A person has a disability for the purposes of the act if he or she has a physical or mental impairment and the impairment has a substantial and long-term adverse effect on his or her ability to carry out normal day-to-day activities.[31] Chapter 7 deals with mental health in depth.

Organisations need to develop an approach to support the health and wellbeing of their employees that completely covers the full range of all employee activities and roles. The Department of Health (2011)[32] stated that the delivery of NHS services involved one of the largest workforces in the world, and that the health and wellbeing of this significant UK workforce were crucial to the delivery of high standards of patient care.

There is strong evidence from the Boorman report[33] to demonstrate that NHS organisations that show commitment to supporting the public health agenda and health and wellbeing programmes for employees reach a positive range of outcomes. The evidence shows that it is clear that cultures of engagement, mutuality, caring, compassion and respect for all (staff, patients and general public) provide the ideal environment within which to care for the health of local populations.

Black set out the national vision for a healthy workforce[34] that would benefit the economy and continue to influence improvements across workforces. In Boorman's review[33] he also suggests that by investing in and prioritising health and wellbeing programmes and the public health agenda, there could be a £555 million productivity improvement realisation by reducing NHS staff sickness absence rates by a third.

The government showed commitment to establishing a culture that supports the reports from Boorman and Black, and the strategy for public health[35] clearly set out that employee health and wellbeing are vital to support staff quality of life, and have a positive impact on the performance of any organisation.

OH nurses have a key role within an organisation to plan and deliver the wellbeing and public health agendas, which in turn will contribute to the business plans of the company. Waddell and Burton[23] suggest that, to make a wellbeing initiative successful, some key elements need to be considered. These include:

- programmes designed to meet employees' needs and values
- senior management buy-in: this has to go beyond mere endorsement to active and visible participation
- programmes aligned to the overall aims and goals of the business
- good communication, both in terms of employees being informed and updated on initiatives, and being consulted on their needs and views on future programmes
- a means of measuring the outcomes and business benefits.

Alongside the OH professionals, the support of human resources (HR), health and safety practitioners and trade union representatives is key for the success of these programmes.

The culture of the organisation needs to be taken into consideration. For instance, investing in a large health promotion programme may not result in sustained health improvement unless the organisation's underpinning health and safety culture is positive, as without this, the programme is likely to have little impact.

It is essential to seek the views of employees and to involve them in the process when it comes to health promotion and wellbeing programmes in the workplace. They are much more likely to be successful with full workforce involvement and helping to identify those health and wellbeing issues that need addressing. More indepth information is given on health promotion in Chapter 4.

Specific programmes to support the public health agenda

One important aspect of wellbeing is around supporting employees with specific health conditions to remain in work or to return in a timelier manner with appropriate support and reasonable adjustments in place.

There has been a belief among some employers that employees with new or ongoing health conditions should not return to work until they are fully fit. However, more recently, and with greater input from OH professionals, this has been shown not to be the case, and actually, an earlier return to work is more beneficial to enable the employee to return to a 'normal' routine. Waddell and Burton support this and highlight the benefits of work in providing the economic stability, social networking and self-esteem that are important for an individual's physical and mental wellbeing. There is increasing awareness, too, that many common health conditions can be effectively managed within the workplace, leading to increased and positive health outcomes and reduced sickness absence.

The OH nurse can therefore be seen to be the key link between the primary care to support existing health conditions, providing the health promotion programmes to support individuals in reducing the risk of developing a new health condition, and the employer to support HR professionals in reducing sickness absence and increasing productivity. The OH nurse needs to focus on the high-profile areas that have been discussed, and are known to have an impact on health, and put programmes in place to support employees who wish to improve or prevent such health conditions.

How would you define mental wellbeing? Consider if any changes in your practice need to be considered to encompass this.

Mental wellbeing

Statistics from the Sainsbury's Centre[36] demonstrate evidence of the considerable costs associated with mental health in the work environment. On average, one in six employees are affected by a mental health condition such as depression, stress or anxiety. This number can be increased to one in five if drug or alcohol dependence is also included. Mental health conditions account for around 40 per cent of sickness absence, which can be broken down to around 3 days per year per employee, and stress and mental ill health may account for up to 5 per cent of employee turnover. Mental health issues are dealt with in depth in Chapter 7.

An effective public health strategy should have a holistic view of mental wellbeing and needs to include the following:

- Legal requirements set out to prevent mental ill health need to be considered. The Health and Safety Executive (HSE)'s stress management standards[37] and the CIPD/HSE/Investors in People stress competency framework[38] provide guidance to OH and other professionals on how to assess the work environment and provide a baseline to measure against.
- Frequent assessment of how the organisation is performing against the HSE management standards will ensure that areas for improvement can be identified by the OH professional and addressed by the employer. It could be argued that the OH nurse or the HR professional should also carry out stress audits or surveys to gain an overall picture of the organisation's stress.
- The OH and HR professionals should ensure that robust recruitment practices are in place to comply with the Equality Act, that applicants with a history of mental health conditions are not discriminated against and that all reasonable adjustments are considered, and ongoing support is available if the new employee requires it.
- Partnership working between health and safety, HR and OH should be discussed to ensure competent training for managers is in place to increase their understanding of mental ill health and mental wellbeing, and their ability and legal responsibilities to support the employee who may have further problems in the future. They need to be able to identify and address the early signs of mental distress and how work can have a negative impact on an individual's wellbeing.
- Employees need to be encouraged to look after their own mental wellbeing. The OH professional can assist by supporting them by providing advice around healthy choices such as a balanced diet and exercise, as these are both good for physical and mental wellbeing, and help to build mental and emotional resilience.

- Organisations need to make provision for access to specialist support and so collaborative working with counsellors and other therapists such as cognitive behavioural therapists should be discussed with senior managers within the organisation to ensure adequate funding and resources are available.
- OH nurses need to ensure comprehensive rehabilitation programmes are in place to assist in the timely return to work, if an employee has required time off sick. Again, collaborative working between the manager, HR and OH is essential to support the employee back to work, taking into consideration any temporary or permanent adjustments to the workplace or role that would help to reduce the chances of a recurrence.

Physical wellbeing

Musculoskeletal disorders (MSDs) such as low-back pain are very common, and even more frequent in organisations such as the NHS. It has been shown that almost half (49 per cent) of the UK's adult population have reported low back pain that has lasted for more than 24 hours at some point in the last 12 months. It can also be said that 80 per cent will experience back pain at some stage in their lives.[39] As well as back pain, it is recognised that some work tasks can lead to employees experiencing upper-limb and neck problems. These work practices often relate to repetitive or prolonged single-action tasks, such as production line working, computer or keyboard work, the use of vibrating tools or poor work environment such as poorly designed workstations. If these problems are not addressed they may lead to permanent health issues. The HSE statistics[40] show that in 2009–2010 an estimated 572,000 employees in the UK suffered from an MSD that was either caused or exacerbated by their work. Of these, 248,000 suffered from back pain, 230,000 from an upper-limb pain, while 94,000 reported a lower-limb issue.

The OH nurse needs to consider all aspects of the condition, and understand that it is often difficult to identify the one single cause. However, with a full and comprehensive assessment, the OH nurse is able to identify the contributing factors which can be:

- a history of back pain
- smoking and obesity
- physical factors such as heavy manual work, frequent bending, twisting, lifting, pulling, pushing, repetitive work or vibration
- other factors, such as stress, anxiety, depression or poor job satisfaction.

With this assessment and close working relations with other professionals such as health and safety advisers, physiotherapists or ergonomists, a physical wellbeing approach includes the following:

- Working with the legal requirements and guidance set out by the HSE to prevent or reduce work-related MSDs: this includes risk assessments, good ergonomics and early intervention by physiotherapists if a problem does occur.

- The OH nurse needs to consider setting up individual plans with the employee to encourage physical activity and fitness. If there is an existing back condition, programmes may need to be tailored to ensure further injury does not occur.
- By working with external agencies such as local gyms, fitness and sports centres or groups, the OH nurse is able to provide information and support to the employee in both prevention and rehabilitation.
- The OH nurse will be involved with the rehabilitation plans for all employees who have been affected by an MSD, whether this is a work or non-work-related injury, as both will have an impact on attendance and productivity in the short, medium and possibly longer term.

Healthy eating and obesity

Research carried out in 2007 shows that obesity in the UK has trebled during the past 25 years.[41] It is also associated with the higher incidence of an individual suffering from a number of chronic illnesses, such as cardiovascular disease, diabetes, certain types of cancers, and joint conditions or disorders. The research suggests that obesity has cost the UK 18 million lost working days and 30,000 deaths each year. This increase in obesity could be seen to be linked mainly to a decrease in physical activity as calorie intake does not appear to have changed since 1980.

Healthy eating is not just about maintaining a healthy weight. A balanced diet can help prevent digestive disorders, iron deficiency, bone conditions such as osteoarthritis, cancers linked to the digestive system and others such as breast cancer that could be linked to hormone-related conditions. Ahrens[42] suggests that deficiencies in minerals and vitamins may be linked to low moods and depression. This needs to be considered as employees with balanced diets and good eating habits may have higher concentration levels, more energy, less absence due to digestive-related issues and ultimately higher performance levels.

With this in mind, the opposite needs to be taken into account, as obesity may have a negative impact on health and safety at work. If an employee's fitness and physical activity is low, then he or she may be more susceptible to injury from manual handling tasks. Even in more sedentary roles, there may be an impact, as standard office equipment may not be suitable for the employee to use.

The OH nurse should consider this aspect of the public health agenda sensitively, as many employees struggle to come forward and ask for help and advice. Health promotion activities should focus on physical fitness and maintaining a healthy and balanced diet. Collaborative work alongside a dietician will assist the employee even further as the dietician will be able to have a greater understanding about food types and the effects on the body.

The OH nurse approach to this aspect of wellbeing is about embedding healthy eating and activity into all aspects of work and the environment. Ensuring the canteen has healthy options available, corporate gym membership, health promotion information available in staff areas such as rest rooms and canteens and the promotion of all activities routinely communicated through staff newsletters and websites all help to offer employees a healthy way of living.

The OH nurse is available to offer support and advice to the employer on how work pressures may have a negative impact on an employee's diet. As part of a health promotion and wellbeing campaign, encouraging employees to take responsibility for preparing healthy food to bring into work, ensuring that they do not skip meals such as breakfast, and that they take time to have a lunch break are all simple steps to healthier living.

Smoking

Smoking has become a worldwide issue, and in the UK this has been reflected in the number of government papers and campaigns that have been delivered to try to tackle this problem. The risks associated with smoking were notably published by Fletcher and Peto in 1977:[43] this has remained a key study which is often quoted in current research. It identified that the risks were mainly linked to early death and respiratory disease.

According to the NHS,[44] smoking is one of the biggest causes of death and illness in the UK, resulting in 114,000 deaths a year. Smoking increases the risk of at least 50 medical conditions, some of which may be fatal whereas others may cause chronic health conditions. These can include cancers of the lung, mouth and throat, coronary heart disease, stroke, emphysema, reduced fertility, dementia and digestive disorders.

By law, all workplaces in the UK must now be smokefree.[45] Employers should have smokefree policies and look at programmes to support employees who wish to quit.

For the OH nurse, there are other aspects to consider as smoking may also exacerbate some work-related conditions, for example, asbestos-related disease, vibration white finger and asthma.

Therefore during a health assessment the OH nurse needs to ensure a full history is taken, and all opportunities to encourage smoking cessation are discussed and offered.

Alcohol and drugs

Alcohol

There are clear work-related health and safety and legal issues in allowing employees to be at work whilst under the influence of alcohol or drugs. Employees affected by alcohol or drugs are likely to demonstrate poorer performance if they are at work and have a higher level of sickness absence.[46]

It is necessary to consider the effect of alcohol or drugs on the workforce as a whole, particularly if one employee has a problem as this may have a negative effect on the rest of the workforce. More than 90 per cent of people in the UK (over the age of 16) drink alcohol. Whereas drinking in moderation is less likely to cause any ill health effects, too much drinking or drinking at the wrong time can be detrimental to health. Over the past three decades, alcohol has become increasingly more available to all and is cheaper. According to the Royal College of Psychiatrists, around 1 in 15 men and 1 in 50 women are physically addicted to alcohol.[47]

Alcohol is a major cause of accidents and injury, and the presence of alcohol in the system has also been proven to increase the severity of any injury.[48] For these reasons, in safety-critical jobs, such as trackside rail workers, consumption of alcohol is very closely monitored and regulated.

In 1979–1980 in the UK, the HSE carried out investigations on work-related fatal incidents and found a blood alcohol level which exceeded the legal drink-drive limit on 35 out of 92 incidents. The HSE estimates that alcohol causes between 3 and 5 per cent of all absences from work, which can be equated to between 8 and 14 million working days lost.

Although alcohol misuse is not classically seen as an OH issue as it is not, in its self, a health condition, the effects on the individual and the safety implications certainly make it a case for the OH nurse to support the employer in ensuring that employees are offered appropriate and specialist treatment and advice and to promote a healthy lifestyle which includes safer levels of alcohol intake.

Drugs

It is an offence, under the Misuse of Drug Act 1971, to produce, supply and possess most controlled drugs except in certain circumstances such as when prescribed by a doctor.

The 2009–2010 British Crime Survey estimates that in 1 year nearly 9 per cent of adults had used illegal drugs and over 3 per cent had used a class A drug.[49]

An HSE report on the impact of illegal drug use by workers[50] found that in a survey, 13 per cent reported using drugs in the previous 12 months; drug use is closely linked to smoking and drinking alcohol. The use of recreational drugs may also affect safety at work.

Employers may have solvents within the workplace as part of the function of the company. OH nurses need to be aware of the potential for misuse and, working closely with the employer in raising drug awareness (including solvent misuse), help write policies and ensure that comprehensive and robust testing facilities are available where necessary. As some companies require testing and screening as part of the terms and conditions of employment, the OH nurse should ensure that this is implemented with care and offer a supportive service.

The OH nurse should always make sure the employer is aware that screening will not provide a solution to a problem, but only serves to highlight if there is a problem that needs to be addressed outside the health setting.

The ageing workforce

The HSE has reported that the physical and mental capabilities of the older workforce vary greatly,[51] and so any adaptations to the work tasks or environment need to be assessed on an individual basis.

Musculoskeletal changes are known to occur in ageing, with a marked decrease in flexibility and muscle weakness, and so the older employee will need to have any manual handling tasks assessed on a more frequent basis. In order to ensure that a full and comprehensive assessment of environment and tasks is taken into consideration to protect the health and safety of older workers, the OH nurse may consider consulting with an ergonomist. It is more likely that factors such as exercise, smoking, lifestyle and diet have a greater impact on health than age, and so health promotion programmes and initiatives set up in the workplace would be of benefit to all employees, irrespective of age.

The employer will recognise that the employee who has been with the organisation for a period of time or within that field of work is likely to have a greater knowledge and skill base which will have a positive effect on productivity. It is therefore suggested that the OH service should offer a full range of health and wellbeing programmes which will cover the public health agenda.

Activity

Review your current health promotion and wellbeing programmes and spend some time looking at your processes and procedures. Consider if they provide employers and employees with appropriate support and advice.

Conclusion

The government has stated that it is committed to improving the health and wellbeing of the UK workforce and to reducing the cost associated with health-related job loss. Preventing employees leaving work due to ill health has to be better than primary care teams having to manage long-standing, chronic conditions with the unemployed. With appropriate and timely interventions by OH, and the support of employers who can accommodate adjustments and provide the resources and facilities to deliver the public health and wellbeing programmes alongside all other streams of OH practice, employees will continue to provide a full and productive service to their employers.

References

1 Viseltear A (1982) Winslow and the early years of public health at Yale, 1915–1925. *Yale Journal of Biological Medicine* 55: 137–150.
2 https://www.gov.uk/government/topics/public-health.
3 Department of Health (2006) *Our Health, Our Care, Our Say: A new direction for community services*. London: Department of Health.
4 Department of Health (2000) *The NHS Plan: A plan for investment, a plan for reform*. London: The Stationery Office.
5 Darzi A (2008) *High Quality Care for All: NHS next stage review*. London: Department of Health.
6 Darzi A (2008) *A High Quality Workforce: NHS next stage review*. London: Department of Health.

7   Darzi A (2008) *NHS Next Stage Review: Our vision for primary and community care*. London: Department of Health.

8   Faculty of Occupational Medicine (2010) *Safe Effective Quality Occupational Health Service: Occupational health service standards for accreditation*. London: Faculty of Occupational Medicine.

9   Department of Health and Social Security (1980) *The Black Report*. London: Department of Health.

10 Acheson D (1998) *Independent Enquiry into Inequalities in Health Report*. London: The Stationery Office.

11 Department of Health (1998) *Our Healthier Nation: A contract for health*. London: Department of Health.

12 Department of Health (1999) *Saving Lives: Our healthier nation*. London: The Stationery Office.

13 Welsh Assembly Government (2002) *Wellbeing in Wales*. Cardiff: Welsh Assembly Government.

14 Scottish Executive (2003) *Improving Health in Scotland: The challenge*. Edinburgh: Scottish Executive.

15 Department of Health, Social Services and Public Safety (2004) *A Healthier Future: A twenty year vision for health and wellbeing in Northern Ireland 2005–2025*. Belfast: Department of Health, Social Services and Public Safety.

16 Scottish Executive (2005) *Delivering for Health*. Edinburgh: Scottish Executive.

17 Scottish Government (2007) *Better Health, Better Care*. Edinburgh: Scottish Government.

18 Department of Health (2002) *Tackling Health Inequalities Through Local Public Service Agreements*. London: Department of Health.

19 Department of Health (2003) *Tackling Health Inequalities: A programme for action*. London: Department of Health.

20 Department of Health (2004) *Choosing Health: Making healthier choices easier*. London: Department of Health.

21 Department of Health (2005) *Delivering Choosing Health: Making healthier choices easier*. London: Department of Health.

22 Marmot review (2010) *Fair Society, Healthy Lives: Post 2010 strategic review of health inequalities*. London: UCL Research Department of Epidemiology and Public Health.

23 Waddell G, Burton K (2006) *Is Work Good for Your Health and Wellbeing?* London: The Stationery Office.

24 Chartered Institute of Personnel and Development (2007) *What's Happening with Wellbeing at Work?* London: CIPD. Available online at: www.cipd.co.uk/hr-resources/research/well-being-at-work.aspx.

25 Department for Work and Pensions, Department of Health and Health and Safety Executive (2005) *Health, Work and Wellbeing – Caring for our future: a strategy for the health and wellbeing of working aged people*. London: Department of Health.

26 Institute of Directors (2006) *Wellbeing at Work: How to manage workplace wellness to boost your staff and business performance*. London: IOD.

27 Black C, Frost D (2011) *Health at Work: An independent review of sickness absence*. London: The Stationery Office.

28 Department of Health (2011) *Public Health Responsibility Deal*. London: Department of Health. Available online at: https://responsibilitydeal.dh.gov.uk/about.

29 Young V, Bhaumik C (2011) *Health and Wellbeing at Work: A survey of employers*. Research report no. 750. London: Department for Work and Pensions.

30 Department for Work and Pensions (2013) *Fitness to Work: The government response to 'Health at Work – An independent review of sickness absence'*. London: The Stationery Office.

31 HM Government (2010) *Equality Act 2010 Guidance: Guidance on matters to be taken into account in determining questions relating to the definition of disability*. London: Office for Disability Issues.

32 Department of Health (2011) *NHS Health and Wellbeing Improvement Framework*. London: Department of Health.

33 Boorman S (2009) *NHS Health and Wellbeing: Final report*. London: Department of Health.

34 Black C (2008) *Working for a Healthier Tomorrow*. London: TSO. Available online at: http://www.dwp.gov.uk/docs/hwwb-working-for-a-healthier-tomorrow.pdf.

35 Department of Health (2010) *Healthy Lives, Healthy People: Our strategy for public health in England*. London: Department of Health.

36 The Sainsbury Centre for Mental Health (2007) *Mental Health at Work: Developing a business case*. Policy paper 8. Available online at: www.scmh.org.uk/pdfs/mental_health_at_work.pdf.

37 Health and Safety Executive (2009) *Management Standards for Work Related Stress*. Available online at: www.hse.gov.uk/stress/standards/index.htm.

38 CIPD (2009) *Line Management Behaviour and Stress at Work*. Available online at: www.cipd.co.uk/hr-resources/guides/line-management-behaviour-stress.aspx.

39 BackCare (2013) *Back Facts*. Available online at: www.backcare.org.uk.

40 Health and Safety Executive (2010) *Health and Safety Statistics 2009/10*. Available online at: www.hse.gov.uk/statistics/overall/hssh0910.pdf.

41 Butland B, Jebb S, Kopelman P, McPherson K, Thomas S, Mardell J, Parry V (2007) *Trends and Drivers of Obesity: A literature review for the Foresight project on obesity*. Available online at: www.bis.gov.uk/assets/bispartners/foresight/docs/obesity/literature_review.pdf.

42 Ahrens U (2006) *Food Facts: Food and mood*. British Dietetic Association. Available online at: www.bda.uk.com/foodfacts/FoodMood.pdf.

43 Fletcher C, Peto R (1977) The natural history of chronic airflow obstruction. *Br Med J* 1: 1645–1648.

44 NHS (undated) *What Are the Health Risks of Smoking?* Available online at: http://www.nhs.uk/chq/Pages/2344.aspx?CategoryID=53.

45 The Smoke-free (Premises and Enforcement) Regulations 2006. Available online at: http://www.legislation.gov.uk/uksi/2006/3368/introduction.

46 http://www.hse.gov.uk/alcoholdrugs.

47 The Royal College of Psychiatrists (2008) *Alcohol and Depression*. Available online at: www.rcpsych.ac.uk.

48 Hoare J, Flatley J (2008) *Drug Misuse Declared: Findings from 2007/8 British Crime Survey*. London: Home Office.

49 Flatley J, Kershaw C, Smith K, Chaplin R, Moon D (2010) *Home Office Statistical Bulletin. Crime in England and Wales 2009/10*. Findings from the British Crime Survey and police recorded crime. London: Home Office.

50 Smith A, Wadsworth E, Moss S, Simpson S (2004) *The Scale and Impact of Illegal Drug Use by Workers*. HSE. Available online at: http://www.hse.gov.uk/research/rrpdf/rr193sum.pdf.

51 Benjamin K, Wilson S (2005) *Facts and Misconceptions about Age, Health Status and Employability*. HSL/2005/20. Buxton: Health & Safety Laboratory. Available online at: http://www.hse.gov.uk/research/hsl_pdf/2005/hsl0520.pdf.

3 Leadership

Christina Butterworth

Learning objectives

After reading this chapter you will be able to:

- discuss the fundamental principles of leadership
- discuss the various leadership styles and models
- appreciate how to develop organisation strategy based on business needs and clinical excellence
- describe the impact of team dynamics and stakeholder engagement on delivering strategy
- describe the interaction between the leader, the team and the organisation.

Leadership in occupational health (OH) nursing is a fundamental requirement if practitioners are to meet the challenges of the changing work environment and ongoing development of professional practice. Leadership is different from management in that it is not process-oriented, but flexible to changing needs of the workplace and the people who come into contact with the activities of OH nurses. It is driven by a long-term vision rather than defined outcomes. Leadership is not defined by a role or title but by action, a clear mission and purpose, supporting behaviours and tangible health improvement. All too often nursing leadership is portrayed negatively with cases in the national media that highlight poor nursing care, including the cases of Beverley Allitt, Mid Staffordshire NHS Hospitals and Winterbourne View Hospital.[1] The Boorman Report[2] also made some key points about the impact of the health and happiness of nurses on the care they provide to their patients and therefore their leadership effectiveness.

Strategic leadership forms part of the Nursing and Midwifery Council (NMC) *Standards of Proficiency for Specialist Community Public Health Nursing*[3] and requires OH nurses to develop leadership skills and manage projects to improve health and wellbeing of individuals and groups.

The leader is often regarded as being the person who is in charge or who manages a team or group of people. The leader sets direction, creates an impelling vision and works with others to achieve the strategic objectives. He or she may have a unique set of technical and business-specific knowledge, skills or experience; he or she may lead the organisation or 'lead' on certain issues. Everyone takes a lead role at some time in their lives and uses the skills they have learnt or their personal characteristics to get the desired results. A good leader will of course have to use management skills at times and these will be covered in Chapter 8.

Leadership means different things to different people and we have all worked with people who have demonstrated both good and poor leadership.

Activity

Think about someone you have worked with in the past who has shown good leadership. What were this person's key attributes? How would you define leadership?

Leadership definition

There are as many definitions of leadership as there are those who seek to find the answer. It depends on the people and the situation. The following examples give a broad range of the meaning of the term.

'A leader shapes and shares a vision which gives point to the work of others' (Charles Handy[4]).

'Leaders are people who do the right things; managers are people who do things right' (Professor Warren G Bennis[5]).

'Leadership may be defined as the capacity to influence people, by means of personal attributes and/or behaviours, to achieve a common goal' (Chartered Institute of Personnel and Development (CIPD)[6]).

It could be concluded that leadership by definition is the ability of a charismatic leader to develop a compelling and shared vision and a set of high-quality actions owned by and benefiting all stakeholders.

Handy's[7] seminal textbook recognised that there were a number of leadership theories and he proposed that a new adaptive model was required to meet the needs of any given group, the tasks they wanted to achieve and the environment in which they were operating, as there is no one-size-fits-all model available.

Leadership theories and models

As stated previously, leadership means different things to different people and the concepts of leadership have developed from trait theories,[8,9,10] where it was thought that good leaders were born with innate leadership characteristics, to encompass a range of theories and models that explore the knowledge, skills and situational awareness required to meet the potential for leadership.

The early trait theories (Galton[9]) focused on defining those characteristics exhibited by effective leaders in comparison to those who were less effective. The characteristics include personality, interests and abilities and were thought to be inherited and not able to be developed. Later theories sought to analyse further these prevailing leadership traits and how they were able to influence in given situations (Zaccaro et al.[8]) or focused on understanding the core personality traits of effective leaders in order to develop potential leaders (Derue et al.[10]).

The majority of the leadership theories have the needs of the organisation and team as a core concept. However, OH nurses also have to consider the additional needs of the profession, in order to achieve clinical effectiveness. Both the NMC Specialist Practitioner standards of proficiency[11] and the Royal College of Nursing guidance on OH nursing career and competencies development have leadership as a core requirement. Continuing professional development (CPD) as required for maintaining nurse registration is one such way to address the development of leadership skills. This is not necessarily restricted to clinical care, as some professionals may think, but includes all forms of study, formal or informal. The NMC requires OH nurses to meet the Prep[12] standards as part of their professional registration, by completing:

- 450 hours of registered practice in the previous 3 years
- 35 hours of learning activity (CPD) in the previous 3 years.

The NMC states that: 'The practice standard can be met through administrative, supervisory, teaching, research and managerial roles as well as providing direct patient care.'

The most comprehensive and contemporary piece of research on the topic and concept that has given people much debate for many years is the research from the Work Foundation.[13] The research has shown the benefits of outstanding leadership to an organisation. Nine themes and three fundamental organising principles were identified (Box 3.1). The aim of the research was to define leadership and additionally determine the attributes of both a good and an outstanding leader.

The first of the fundamental organising principles focused on thinking and acting strategically. The OH nurse is required not only to recognise and appreciate all of the individual elements that make up an effective service, but also to step back and appreciate the full picture in terms of people, purpose and interactions. All the research suggests that to be a leader requires confidence, team cohesion and empowerment, trusting the team to do the right things and do them right, creativity, efficient problem solving and being politically astute. Leaders need to recognise who their stakeholders are, how to influence their perception of needs and their commitment to the present strategy and plan and what is potentially required, in the case of OH, for the sustainable delivery of good health provision for the future.

Box 3.1   Nine themes and three organising principles of outstanding leadership

Outstanding leaders think and act systematically

1. Think systematically and act long-term – vision
2. Bring meaning to life
3. Apply the spirit, not the letter of the law
4. Grow people through performance
5. Are self-aware and authentic to leadership first, their own needs second
6. Understand that talk is work
7. Give time and space to others
8. Put 'we' before 'me'
9. Take deeper breaths and hold them longer

Themes

- Outstanding leaders thinking and acting systematically
- Outstanding leaders perceive relationships as the route to performance
- Outstanding leaders achieve through their impact on others

Source: Tamkin P, Pearson G, Hirsh W, Constable S (2010) *Exceeding Expectations: The principles of outstanding leadership*. London: The Work Foundation. Available online at: http://www.theworkfoundation.com/Assets/Docs/leadershipFINAL_reduced.pdf (accessed 26.03.11).

The second principle focuses on relationships and why it is important to spend time on building and maintaining strong and effective relationships within the team and organisation to achieve outstanding performance. An OH nurse leader is already in a strong position to demonstrate this, as relationships are at the core of their work. The relationships within OH nursing span from 'caring' for the individuals for whom they provide clinical care, supporting the organisation they work for and working with its stakeholders to meet business needs. This principle also recognises that the concept of a singular leader with many followers is just that, a concept, for a good leader will by default create fellow leaders, those who aspire to be the future leader in the organisation or a subset thereof.

The third principle focuses on the leader's impact on others. Having self-awareness and recognising that the end goal is health excellence, not the performance of an individual but through individuals. The key role of the leader is to act as a conduit through which the leader influences others to support the vision and focus efforts to achieve the end goal. The OH nurse leader will work to build competence in the team and organisation and create opportunities to step back on occasion to see that they are going in the right direction.

A review of the principles above by Harriss and Witwicka's research[14] concluded that, though the key themes were relevant to OH practice, it would be difficult for OH nurses to achieve outstanding leadership due to the prevailing economic climate and expectations of client groups and stakeholders. If OH nurses truly are to lead then this is exactly why they need to adopt the key characteristics, skills and principles to meet the challenges of working in the new global business world and achieving their vision.

Leadership styles and models

> Leadership style can be defined as a stable mode of behaviour that the leader uses in his and her effort to increase his or her influence, which constitutes the essence of leadership. 'A leader's style refers to the characteristics which are most typical across situations.'[15]

There is a plethora of material on different leadership styles and models that can be readily found with minimal research and this chapter seeks to focus on four main groups of leadership styles and models: trait, behavioural, contingency and power. Good leaders adapt their style to suit the differing circumstances, the social, political and cultural environment of the organisation and the desired outcomes. There are advantages and disadvantages within each leadership style and, to help become an effective leader, knowledge of these various styles will help in matching the style to the situation.

Trait leadership

Trait leadership was developed from early research[10] on patterns of the inherited characteristics of leaders in comparison to those who were not considered to be leaders. The theory[16] focused on what made leaders effective and included traits such as confidence, assertiveness, decision making, problem solving, integrity, charisma and openness. This theory has been challenged due to the premise that leadership is more about nature than nurture and not a true indicator of effectiveness.[17] Research on trait leadership continues because of its potential application in the development of leadership training and for the selection of future leaders. The Big Five[18] personality traits are the most commonly used to describe human personality and to assess performance.[18] Poropat identified some commonly recurring personality traits and grouped them into the Big Five factors. These are openness, conscientiousness, extraversion, agreeableness and neuroticism and are used to describe human personality. No single or multiple traits can predict success as a leader but they do help to identify qualities that will help OH nurses lead effectively.

Behavioural leadership

Theories on behavioural styles emerged as a response to the early criticisms of the trait approach and focused on the patterns of behaviours that effective leaders exhibited and how they could be learned and developed.

Kurt Lewin's[19] seminal work in the 1930s on behavioural-based leadership styles and performance argued that there are three types of behavioural leadership styles: autocratic, participative and laissez-faire.

Autocratic leadership

The autocratic leadership style allows managers to make all the decisions. Managers have total authority and dominate team members. No one challenges the decisions and this style results in one or two cases of passive resistance from some team members and yet benefits those team members who need close supervision and direction from the leader. This style may be effective in getting urgent action completed and does appeal to some team members but it stifles creative employees and those who want some decision-making ability.

Participative leadership

Often called the democratic leadership style, participative leadership values the input of team members and peers, but the control over decision making still rests with the leader. Participative leadership involves consultation with team members and joint decision making, thus boosting employee morale. Ownership of the decision is shared and team members feel as if their opinions matter. The leader recognises and uses the strengths of the team members, delegates some responsibility and values group discussions to gain maximum performance but never fails to take full responsibility for leadership. The leader acts as a guide in the decision-making process, allowing greater participation and building trust. This style is effective during organisation change and when decision making is needed quickly.

Laissez-faire leadership

A laissez-faire leadership style is a hands-off approach where the leader encourages the team members to work without direct supervision. Individual decision making and problem solving are encouraged and this benefits those team members who are highly competent and have shown that they can produce high-quality work. The leader tends to have little control over the work activities and just provides advice and support to team members when needed. However, not all team members are able to work autonomously and may need some direction and motivation. This approach can lead to poor outcomes in terms of production, resource allocation and increasing costs.

OH nurses should consider how their behavioural style as a manager affects their relationship with the teams they work with and how the choice in style can promote commitment and contribution to the organisational goals and their professional development.

If the required leadership outcome is production, any of the styles is effective. If the criterion is group freedom, the more democratic styles are effective. If fast decision making is the criterion, the styles maximising leader authority seem the best.

Contingency leadership

Following on from the theories of trait and behaviour it became evident that leadership style needed to be flexible and adaptive to the given situation and so contingency theories were developed.

There are a number of popular contingency or situational theories. Fiedler's contingency model[20] suggests that leadership effectiveness depends on both leadership style (being task- or human-oriented) and the degree to which the situation gives the leader control and influence. Three factors affecting a leader's control and influence are identified:

1. the relationship between the leader and followers, whereby support may more easily be gained by a liked and respected leader
2. the structure of the task, whereby clarity of the goals, methods and criteria will promote greater influence
3. the leader's positional power, which may afford the leader greater control.

Hersey–Blanchard Situational Leadership Theory[21] also focuses on the leadership style and links this with the maturity of the individual members of the team.

OH nursing is dynamic and no two days are the same, with a mixture of medical assessments, research, management system development, audit and risk management all requiring a degree of leadership. Therefore the leadership style adopted by the OH nurse will differ depending on the situation, for example, if you need a quick decision following an incident or when the team needs to pull together to get a project completed or when team members are going through a period of unplanned change. Knowing which style to use depends on the knowledge, understanding and personal experience of the OH nurse.

Transactional and transformational leadership

Burns, in his book *Leadership,*[22] distinguished two types of power leadership: transactional and transformational.

Transactional leadership

Transactional leadership is a leadership style that uses power and influence over the team or task to succeed.

The transactional leader has certain tasks to perform and is given power to lead the team to achieve the agreed goals. The leader is able to monitor and evaluate the performance of the team members in order to train and instruct them and where necessary correct the work if it does not meet the required standard. The team members follow the leader and will be rewarded or punished depending on the performance results.

In OH nursing this leadership style can be used to ensure compliance with clinical standards and to meet expectations on how activities are completed in any given business environment.

Transformational leadership

Transformational leadership is based on the sharing of a vision which motivates and directs the team members. This theory was further extended by Bass[23] to recognise the impact of the team and how it transforms the team members to achieve more, to create a sense of identity and to emulate the leader.

Research[24] on transformational leadership has resulted in the introduction of four elements:

1. Individualised consideration – leaders recognise the individual development needs of the team members and act as a mentor coach to the team members. They provide time and space to listen to the follower's concerns and needs, challenge appropriately and seek contribution. The leader gives empathy and support, keeps communication open and respects the input from the team members. Team members aspire to grow and have a deep-seated motivation to achieve.
2. Intellectual stimulation – leaders encourage free thinking and creativity, challenging organisational norms and covert innovation. They nurture and develop people who think independently. The leader believes in lifelong learning and that challenges or barriers are opportunities to create value. Continuous improvement is recognised and followers seek new ways of work.
3. Inspirational motivation – leaders have a strong vision for the future that is appealing and inspiring to followers. Leaders use persuasive language to motivate followers by articulating the need for high standards, communicating optimism about potential achievement of individuals and the team, and encouraging full participation. The leader uses engaging, powerful, clear and detailed communications to engage with the team members. A real sense of meaning and purpose provides the impetus that drives a group forward.
4. Idealised influence – leaders are held in high personal regard due to their high standards of moral and ethical conduct.

OH nurses who adopt a transformational leadership style value the power of communication and are highly visible. They have the end in mind and work with the team members to achieve a shared vision, through manageable goals. The leader and team members are both transformed by the interaction and accomplishment.

The most effective leadership style depends on the interaction between the leader, team members and the situation. Therefore the value of the leadership style is evaluated by the desired outcomes. Leadership style can be learned.

Activity

Use one of the self-assessment tools below to assess your leadership style:

http://www.leadershipacademy.nhs.uk/discover/leadership-framework-self-assessment-tool

http://www.mindtools.com/pages/article/newLDR_50.htm

Developing organisational strategy

The effective leader creates a compelling vision or mission which then needs to be developed into a tangible strategy and plan. The OH strategy, like any other business strategy, seeks to achieve a particular goal or set of goals and should be based on the needs of all stakeholders – organisation, profession and clients.

Definition of a strategy

> the determination of the basic long-term goals and objectives of an enterprise, and the adoption of courses of action and the allocation of resources necessary for carrying out these goals.
>
> (Chandler[25])

There is more than one format, but all strategic planning needs to go through a systematic process to determine if a formal plan is required. The classic four-step approach to strategic planning[26] is a simple structure to develop and implement a strategic plan:

- Step 1: Where are we now?
- Step 2: Where do we want to get to?
- Step 3: How are we going to get there?
- Step 4: How will we know when we have got there?

Step 1: Where are we now? Situation analysis

In this stage the context in which the strategy is being developed is analysed. A detailed assessment of key factors in the organisation, the field of OH and the health profile of the population being cared for should be conducted.

An organisation assessment should include: gathering information about the structure and culture of the organisation, its commitment to OH in the past and potential for the future, the financial position, changes and success of present or past strategies, views of stakeholders and the governance structure in which the OH service operates. An assessment of the external environment using political, economic, social, technological, environmental, legal and industry (PESTELI)[27] analysis may also be beneficial.

Conducting a benchmarking exercise will help in determining good practice as a yardstick for future performance. The format of the benchmark exercise can range from a simple questionnaire survey to structured interview and review of documentation and practice.

The most widely used tool for the assessment of the present situation is the SWOT analysis to analyse formally the strengths, weaknesses, opportunities and threats. The exercise involves the team brainstorming each of the four elements (Box 3.2).

Box 3.2   SWOT analysis

Internal forces	External forces
Strengths What are we good at?	**Opportunities** Anything happening outside which might actually benefit us if we take advantage of it?
Weaknesses What do we need to get a grip on?	**Threats** Anything happening outside which we need to be able to defend ourselves from?

Source: Schmidt JC, Laycock M (2011) *Understanding the Theory and Process of Strategy Development: Theories of strategic planning.* Available online at: http://www.health knowledge.org.uk/public-health-textbook/organisation-management/5d-theory-process-strategy-development/strategic-planning.

At the end of the SWOT analysis, there should be agreement on how much the organisation has accomplished, what it set out to do, and how it measures up in terms of resources, structure and delivery of the desired outcomes.

The OH nurse should also conduct a health needs assessment to review systematically the health issues facing a population and provide valuable data on gaps in health needs. There are a number of tools[28,29] available that provide a framework for assessment and help to build up a picture of health in the organisation. The benefits of the assessment are to provide evidence about the health of a population and an opportunity to engage with stakeholders and to seek feedback that will help to shape the health strategy.

Step 2: Where do we want to get to? Future direction

This is the development of the vision and strategic objectives. In a large organisation, there is usually an overall vision, and the OH vision has to align to that vision to gain the necessary buy-in. The vision defines the desired or intended future state of a specific organisation in terms of strategic objectives and should meet the SMART test: it should be specific, measurable, achievable, relevant, time-bound.

This step aims to assist stakeholders reach a common understanding by simplifying a large number of ideas into a clear statement and to motivate team members to take action in a chosen direction as efficiently as possible.

Step 3: How are we going to get there? Strategy development

The strategic plan provides a roadmap to get the OH nurse from the present situation to the vision for the future. The format of the strategic plan is flexible and should mirror those already used in the organisation. The project/stakeholder team will come together to review steps 1 and 2 and then draft the strategic plan, which will be a series of programmes. The programmes will have a lead person, team members, desired outcomes, tools, resources and a timeline.

The strategy is likely to be made up of a series of programmes that maintain the present services/products, further develop and grow present programmes or conclude programmes that are no longer required for the new strategy.

Step 4: How will we know when we have got there? Monitoring and evaluation

Once the strategic plan is ready to be put into place a set of monitoring points or milestones are required to check how the plan is progressing. To ensure that this is effective a number of relevant key performance indicators will evaluate the success factors for the plan.

Therefore the OH strategy provides a high-level guide and links activity with the resources needed to achieve it, including: time, money, facilities, environment and skills. Though the strategy may be good and well executed, it does not guarantee success due to unforeseen organisation circumstances and should be reviewed following any major change.

The NHS Leadership Academy's *Leadership Framework*[30] provides a more detailed model that sets out the standard for leadership to which all staff in health and care should aspire. The model is made up of seven domains. Within each domain there are four categories, called elements, and each of these elements is further divided into four descriptors. These statements describe the leadership behaviours which are underpinned by the relevant knowledge, skills and attributes all staff should be able to demonstrate radiating out from those of the individual to those within the wider system.

The five core domains are:

1. Demonstrating personal qualities – effective leadership requires individuals to draw upon their values, strengths and abilities to deliver high standards of service. This requires them to demonstrate effectiveness in developing self-awareness, managing themselves, continuing personal development and acting with integrity.
2. Working with others – effective leadership requires individuals to work with others in teams and networks to deliver and improve services. This requires them to demonstrate effectiveness in developing networks, building and maintaining relationships, encouraging contribution and working within teams.
3. Managing services – effective leadership requires individuals to focus on the success of the organisation(s) in which they work. This requires them to be effective in planning and managing resources, people and performance.
4. Improving services – effective leadership requires individuals to make a real difference to people's health by delivering high-quality services and by developing improvements to services. This requires them to demonstrate effectiveness in ensuring patient safety, critically evaluating, encouraging improvement and innovation and facilitating transformation.

5. Setting direction – effective leadership requires individuals to contribute to the strategy and aspirations of the organisation and act in a manner consistent with its values. This requires them to demonstrate effectiveness in identifying the contexts for change, applying knowledge and evidence, making decisions and evaluating impact.

There are two additional domains which apply particularly, but not exclusively, to individuals in senior leadership roles.

6. Creating the vision – those in senior leadership roles create a compelling vision for the future, and communicate this within and across organisations. This requires them to demonstrate effectiveness in developing the vision for the organisation, influencing the vision of the wider healthcare system, communicating the vision and embodying the vision.

7. Delivering the strategy – those in senior leadership roles deliver the strategic vision by developing and agreeing strategic plans and ensuring that these are translated into achievable operational plans. This requires them to demonstrate effectiveness in framing, developing, implementing and embedding the strategy.

The OH strategy aims to develop both operational and clinical excellence in order to maintain or improve health at work. Chapter 9 provides more details on evidence-based practice and how to apply it to the needs of the organisation.

Strategic delivery

Successful delivering of the OH strategy needs a combination of effective team leadership and stakeholder engagement. Team leadership can be achieved if the leader has a greater understanding of the dynamics of how teams develop and how to manage the potential issues associated with team working.

Team dynamics

Katzenbach[31] defined a team as follows: 'A team is a small number of people with complementary skills who are committed to a common purpose, performance goals and approach for which they hold themselves mutually accountable.'

The make-up and interaction of team members can determine the success or otherwise of the strategic plan. Frank LaFasto and Carl Larson[32] identified five dynamics to fundamental success of a team:

1. The team member: effective team members are those who are experienced, have problem-solving ability, are open to addressing the problem and are action-oriented.
2. Team relationships: the team must be able to give and receive feedback and work together for the good of the overall strategic objective.
3. Team problem solving: an effective team needs a clear and specific goal. They need open and honest communication to create an environment where team members feel comfortable, relaxed and accepting.

4. Team leadership: effective team leadership depends on leadership competencies. A competent leader is focused on the goal, ensures a collaborative climate, builds confidence of team members, sets priorities, demonstrates sufficient 'know-how' and manages performance through feedback.
5. Organisational environment: the climate and culture of the organisation must be conducive to team behaviour.

Teams do not become effective decision makers solely on the fact that they have a shared goal. Bruce Tuckman[33] proposed the four-stage model of team building – forming, storming, norming and performing – which has become the basis for subsequent models.

Forming

In the first stage of team building, the forming of the team takes place. Team members are getting to know each other, the task and what skills they have that may help with the success of the task. They do not want to cause any conflict so avoid strong feelings and just go through the task actions. This stage is usually short and comfortable and the team members have a high level of agreement, whilst determining their own individual needs and expectations.

The forming stage provides the leader with an opportunity to see how individual team members work and how they respond to each other and the task at hand.

Storming

As the group enters the storming stage they start to compete with each other to get their ideas heard. As the tasks become more defined the team members start to confront each other's ideas and thoughts, the full extent of the work is realised and some members may become overwhelmed. Other members may feel that without the full support of all team members the success of the team is hampered.

The storming stage is necessary to the growth of the team and needs careful control by the leader. The behaviours and emotions need to be normalised and focus should be on the decision-making process and the end goal.

Norming

The norming stage is focused around one goal and strategic objective. Team members know each other better and take responsibility for the team and project as a whole, giving up on their own needs. The team ask each other for feedback and recognise the progress established under the present leadership.

There is often a prolonged overlap between storming and norming behaviour. As new tasks come up, the team may lapse back into typical storming-stage behaviour, but this eventually dissipates.

Performing

The performing stage is only reached when teams start to work effectively together. New members may join the team but this does not usually affect the team dynamic. The team leader is able to delegate more of the tasks and the team members feel more able to work together without leadership direction.

Team members may challenge within the new social norm. Even high-performing teams will occasionally revert to the storming stage if they go through significant change.

These stages of team development are all necessary and inevitable in order for the team to grow, solve problems, support each other through challenges and deliver the strategic plan. This model has become the basis for subsequent models.

Lencioni[34] describes the many pitfalls that teams face as they seek to 'row together' by use of storytelling. Even well-intentioned teams sometimes struggle to work together or achieve the strategy and Lencioni reveals five dysfunctions and how to overcome the issues and perform effectively.

The five dysfunctions are:

1. Absence of trust – the team members are unable to understand and open up to one another. They are not willing to show any weaknesses, admit their mistakes or show any concerns about their ability or those of others to achieve the goals. Without a foundation of trust the team will ultimately fail or delay the success of the strategy.
2. Inattention to results – team members or working groups focus on their own achievement and not the team's collective results. This weakens the effectiveness of the team and the potential of the strategy.
3. Fear or conflict – the foundation of trust and commitment to the end results can result in an environment of fear or conflict. Teams need to be open and honest about their fears and concerns so that the team can work through the issues without anyone becoming harmed by the experience or potentially sabotaging the outcomes.
4. Lack of commitment – if team members fail to adopt real commitment to the strategy they will continue to seek self-reward. They need to be able to share their opinions and feel they have been listened to in order to commit to the shared goals.
5. Avoidance of accountability – once the team members have achieved buy-in and commitment they then have to hold each other to account. Strategic plans do not always go to plan and difficult conversations are sometimes required between the leader and the accountable team member. Failure to hold one another accountable creates an environment where avoidance can thrive.

Stakeholder engagement

Stakeholders are people or organisations who are likely to be affected by your activities/ plans or who have a vested interest and could have an impact on the effectiveness of your desired outcomes.

Stakeholder engagement is the collaboration of stakeholders throughout a process in order to gain understanding and intellectual input into the strategy as well as engaging on an emotional, mutual-benefit perspective.

Working in OH requires the OH nurse to engage with a wide variety of stakeholders from team members to senior management, third-party service providers, clients and allied professionals. In order to develop and deliver the OH strategy effectively a stakeholder mapping exercise will help to determine who to involve and to what extent they should be involved and to agree the intended outcomes. Developing long-term strategic partnerships and relationships will support the long-term vision for OH. Not all stakeholders have the same level of input or importance.

Mind Tools[35] recognise the stakeholder planning is critical to the success of every project in every organisation and will provide tangible benefits in the form of shaping the project/strategy, securing resources, supporting the outcomes and ensuring success through the anticipation of other people's reactions. The tool they provide takes you through three steps in analysing stakeholders:

1. Identify your stakeholders – using a brainstorming exercise the leader with the support of others will identify who might be affected by the project/strategy, have power/influence over it or have a vested interest in its success.
2. Prioritise your stakeholders, using a power/interest grid to classify the stakeholders identified in step 1. Where people are placed on the grid determines the actions to take with them in terms of involvement.
3. Understand your key stakeholders – a set of key questions is used to understand how they might feel about the project/strategy and how best to communicate with them.

Stakeholder analysis provides you with the information to engage with those people who can help or hinder the success of your strategy. Though the OH strategy may change the relationships you build with stakeholders will provide long-term gain either directly or indirectly by your reputation as a leader.

Stakeholder engagement is not easy and Hardman and Nichols[36] recognised the problems of getting people to engage, understand and act with the strategy. Using the cascade model of strategy development and implementation creates gaps in both understanding and engagement. Stakeholders need to be able to see the connection between the strategy and what it means on a day-to-day basis. It needs to be logical, motivating and with clear benefits. Not all stakeholders will engage with the process/strategy from the start but these mavericks still need to be involved as they can provide valuable insight into the opportunities and risks in the prevailing environment. The level of engagement does vary and it is important that stakeholders are aware of their role as critical friends in the strategy which may or may not include decision making. Finally, once the strategy is implemented it needs regular review and refinement to meet the changing needs of the organisation.

The benefits of good health at work are well recognised but without the collaboration of those who would benefit the most from the OH strategy it will not be as effective as it could be.

Two reviews,[37,38] conducted by the King's Fund, looked at engagement and leadership in the NHS. The reports recognised that engagement with staff and patients was essential if change was to be successful. Engaged staff deliver better patient care with a direct correlation between patient care and outcomes in terms of errors, infections and mortality rates. The prevailing leadership style was challenged, with a move away from the remit of a few individuals to a more inclusive and prolific domain of people throughout the organisation. The report also recognised that objectives cannot be achieved in isolation.

As the NHS is one of the largest employers in the UK the lessons learnt from the reviews and the recommendation made can easily be transferred to smaller organisations.

Identify the role of teams and individuals in the delivery of the business plan, whilst managing internal and external political environments.

Leader, team and organisation

The OH nurse will need to work to combine the key elements of success: the leader, team and organisation. The OH nurse has an interdependent relationship with mutual dependence of each element focusing on the vision for optimal health at work. The relationship between the leader and the team is task and people development. The leader is not always the manager of the team members but, working on the delivery of the strategy, provides discretionary development of the team members by participating in the plan. The relationship between the organisation and the leader is the impact of the strategy on health performance or the effect of health on work and work on health. The relationship between the team and the organisation is mutual benefit in terms of money, values and end product, health of employees and delivering against the business plan.

Peter Drucker,[39] one of the best-known contemporary management theorists, believes that consistency is the key to good leadership, and that successful leaders share the following three abilities which are based on what he refers to as good old-fashioned hard work:

1. To define and establish a sense of mission. Good leaders set goals, priorities and standards, making sure that these objectives are not only communicated but maintained.
2. To accept leadership as a responsibility rather than a rank. Good leaders aren't afraid to surround themselves with talented, capable people; they do not blame others when things go wrong.
3. To earn and keep the trust of others. Good leaders have personal integrity and inspire trust among their followers; their actions are consistent with what they say.

In Drucker's words, 'Effective leadership is not based on being clever, it is based primarily on being consistent.'

Very simply put, leading is establishing direction and influencing others to follow that direction. Keep in mind that no list of leadership traits and skills is definitive because no two successful leaders are alike. What is important is that leaders exhibit some positive characteristics that make them effective managers at any level in an organisation.

Conclusion

OH nurses work in a wide variety of organisations, each with individual needs and priorities, and can work in small, medium or large teams, as well as on their own. The environment in which OH nurses work and how they interact with other OH and non-OH professionals mean that the OH nurse needs to demonstrate leadership skills in order to deliver operational and professional excellence. This chapter has considered how the knowledge of leadership theory and styles can provide the OH nurse with a range of approaches to different leadership situations. It has also considered the need to create a compelling vision and engage with stakeholders in the organisation to develop and deliver a health strategy which is aligned with the needs of the organisation and profession. It is not possible to cover every aspect of this vast topic in one chapter but the references and web links should lead you to further and indepth reading of this subject as well as a number of useful tools. Effective leaders can add value simply by being present on teams. They do not need to be the senior manager within the organisation and can show leadership in self-directed work tasks and small-group work, in an inspirational and motivating manner. Develop these leadership skills in yourself and in your team members, and you'll see improvements in health at work.

References

1 Department of Health (2012) *Transforming Care: A national response to Winterbourne View Hospital: Department of Health review final report*. Available online at: https://www.gov.uk/government/uploads/system/uploads/attachment_data/file/127310/final-report.pdf.pdf.

2 Department of Health (2009) *The Boorman Report: NHS health and well being review, final report*. London: Department of Health.

3 Nursing and Midwifery Council (2004) *Standards of Proficiency for Specialist Community Public Health Nursing*. London: Nursing and Midwifery Council.

4 Handy C (1992) The language of leadership. In: Syrett M, Hogg C (eds) *Frontiers of Leadership*. Oxford: Blackwell.

5 Bennis WG (2009) *On Becoming a Leader*. Reading, MA: Addison-Wesley, p. 67.

6 Chartered Institute of Personnel Development (2012) *Factsheet: Leadership*. Available online at: http://www.cipd.co.uk/hr-resources/factsheets/leadership.aspx.

7 Handy C (1976) *Understanding Organisations*. Middlesex: Penguin, Chapter 4.

8 Zaccaro SJ, Kemp C, Bader P (2004) Leader traits and attributes. In: Antonakis J, Cianciolo AT, Sternberg RJ (eds) *The Nature of Leadership*. Thousand Oaks, CA: Sage Publications, pp. 101–124.

9 Galton F (1869) *Hereditary Genius*. New York: Appleton.

10 Derue DS, Nahrgang JD, Wellman N, Humphrey SE (2011) Trait and behavioral theories of leadership: An integration and meta-analytic test of their relative validity. *Personnel Psychol* 4: 7–52.

11 NMC (2004) *Standards of Proficiency for Specialist Community Public Health Nurses*. London: NMC.

12 NMC (2011) *The Prep Handbook*. London: NMC.

13 Tamkin P, Pearson G, Hirsh W, Constable S (2010) *Exceeding Expectations: The principles of outstanding leadership.* London: The Work Foundation. Available online at: http://www.theworkfoundation.com/Assets/Docs/leadershipFINAL_reduced.pdf (accessed 26.03.11).

14 Harriss A, Witwicka S (2012) A sharper leading edge. *Occup Health* 64 (10): 19–21.

15 Nicolaou-Smokoviti L (2004) Business leaders' work environment and leadership style. *Curr Sociol* 52 (3): monograph 1.

16 Zaccaro SJ (2007) Trait-based perspectives of leadership. *Am Psychologist* 62(1): 6–16.

17 Kenny DA, Zaccaro SJ (1983) An estimate of variance due to traits in leadership. *J Appl Psychol* 68(4): 678–685.

18 Poropat AE (2009) A meta-analysis of the five-factor model of personality and academic performance. *Psychological Bull* 135: 322–338.

19 Lewin K, Lippitt R, White R (1939) Patterns of aggressive behavior in experimentally created social climates. *J Social Psychol* 10: 271–301.

20 Fiedler FE (1967) *A Theory of Leadership Effectiveness.* New York: McGraw-Hill: Harper and Row.

21 Hersey P, Blanchard KH (1977) *Management of Organizational Behavior,* 3rd edn. *Utilizing Human Resources.* New Jersey: Prentice Hall.

22 Burns JM (1978) *Leadership.* New York: Harper and Row.

23 Bass BM (1985) *Leadership and Performance.* New York: Free Press.

24 Bass BM, Bass R (2008) *The Bass Handbook of Leadership: Theory, research, and managerial applications,* 4th edn. New York: Free Press.

25 Chandler AD (1962) *Strategy and Structure.* Cambridge, MA: MIT Press.

26 Schmidt JC, Laycock M (undated) *Understanding the Theory and Process of Strategy Development: Theories of strategic planning.* Available online at: http://www.health knowledge.org.uk/public-health-textbook/organisation-management/5d-theory-process-strategy-development/strategic-planning.

27 Chartered Institute of Personnel Development (2010) *Factsheet: PESTLE analysis.* Available online at: http://www.cipd.co.uk/hr-resources/factsheets/pestle-analysis.aspx.

28 Alchemy for Managers. *An Occupational Health Needs Assessment.* Available online at: http://www.alchemyformanagers.co.uk/topics/7gM53CgBqF3v5s4z.html.

29 *NICE (2005) Building Blocks for a Healthier Workplace: Health needs assessment.* Available online at: http://www.nice.org.uk/aboutnice/whoweare/aboutthehda/hdapub lications/health_needs_assessment_a_practical_guide.jsp.

30 NHS Leadership Academy (2011). *Leadership Framework.* Available online at: http://www.leadershipacademy.nhs.uk/discover/leadership-framework.

31 Katzenbach JR, Smith DK (1993) *The Wisdom of Teams: Creating the high-performance organisations.* Boston, MA: Harvard Business School Press.

32 LaFasto FMJ, LC (2001) *When Teams Work Best.* Thousand Oaks, CA: Sage.

33 Tuckman B (1965) Developmental sequence in small groups. *Psychol Bull* 63 (6): 384–399.

34 Lencioni P (2002) *The Five Dysfunctions of a Team.* San Francisco, CA: Jossey-Bass.

35 Mind Tools (undated) *Stakeholder Analysis: Winning support for your projects.* Available online at: http://www.mindtools.com/pages/article/newPPM_07.htm.

36 Hardman P, Nichols C (2011) Engage – the secret to strategy success. *HR Magazine Most Influential,* September. Available online at: http://www.hrmostinfluential.co.uk/research/engage--the-secret-to-strategy-success (accessed 13.07.13).

37 King's Fund (2012) *Leadership and Engagement for Improvement in the NHS: Together we can.* Report from the King's Fund Leadership Review 2012. London: King's Fund.

38 King's Fund (2011) *Commission on Leadership: No more heroes*. London: King's Fund.
39 Drucker PF (2007) *The Practice of Management*. New York: Harper and Row.

Further reading

Covey SR (2004) *The Seven Habits of Highly Effective People*. New York: Simon & Schuster. This book explains how perception of effectiveness and how it is governed and communicated affect the way we behave and achieve personal and interpersonal effectiveness.

Health promotion and health needs assessment

Siân Edwards

Learning objectives

After reading this chapter you will be able to:

- demonstrate an understanding of the principles of health promotion
- apply the principles of health promotion to the workplace/occupational setting
- appreciate the principles of health needs assessment especially as applied to the occupational setting
- critically evaluate the role of the occupational health (OH) nurse in health promotion.

Introduction

Chapter 1 started with the definition of nursing from the International Council of Nurses:[1]

> Nursing encompasses autonomous and collaborative care of individuals of all ages, families, groups and communities, sick or well and in all settings. Nursing includes the promotion of health, prevention of illness, and the care of ill, disabled and dying people. Advocacy, promotion of a safe environment, research, participation in shaping health policy and in patient and health systems management, and education are also key nursing roles.

Health promotion is therefore a key aspect of nursing in general. Whitaker and Baranski[2] make it quite clear that health promotion is one of the primary roles of the OH nurse in the prevention of occupational injury and disease, the improvement of environmental health and the promotion of health and work ability, by focusing on non-occupational, work-place preventable conditions that, whilst not caused directly by work, may affect the employee's ability to maintain attendance or performance at work, through a comprehensive workplace health promotion strategy.

(p. 25)

Several other authors also include health promotion as a main function of OH nursing.[3,4,5]

Before we continue, it is worth revisiting what we mean by the terms health and health promotion as understanding and recognising individual views and concepts will help in identifying health promotion needs and in designing appropriate health promotion interventions. The World Health Organization (WHO) definition of health is a positive view of health which has been unchanged since 1948; it states that 'health is a state of complete physical, mental and social well-being and not merely the absence of disease or infirmity'.[6] A more recent definition which finds its roots in the WHO is that health is a resource for living rather than an end in itself.[7] Naidoo and Wills[8] use a holistic model of health which encompasses the individual (physical, mental, emotional, spiritual and sexual health) as well as the societal, environmental and global factors affecting health. They also discuss several theories, models and definitions of health and have streamlined them into four main concepts:

1. health as an ideal state
2. health as mental and physical fitness
3. health as a commodity
4. health as a personal strength.

Meanwhile, health promotion has variously been defined as:

- 'promoting healthy living'[4]
- 'comprising effort to enhance positive health and reduce the risk of ill health through the overlapping spheres of health education, prevention and health protection'[9]
- 'Health promotion refers to efforts to prevent ill health and promote positive health. From a relatively narrow focus on changing people's behaviour, health promotion has become a broad and complex field encompassing policy change and community action. The central aim is to enable and empower people to take control of their own health.'[10]
- 'the process of enabling people to increase control over and to protect their health (including providing information about health choices and the effects of poor choices, helping people to set goals and encouraging them to make positive changes for their health).'[11]
- 'contemporary health promotion involves more than simply educating individuals about healthy practices. It includes efforts to change organisational behaviour, as

well as the physical and social environment of communities . . . health promotion programmes that seek to address health problems across the spectrum employ a range of strategies and operate on multiple levels.'[12]

The WHO *Ottawa Charter* in 1986 defined health promotion thus:[13]

Health promotion is the process of enabling people to increase control over, and to improve, their health. To reach a state of complete physical, mental and social well-being, an individual or group must be able to identify and to realize aspirations, to satisfy needs, and to change or cope with the environment. Health is, therefore, seen as a resource for everyday life, not the objective of living. Health is a positive concept emphasizing social and personal resources, as well as physical capacities. Therefore, health promotion is not just the responsibility of the health sector, but goes beyond healthy lifestyles to well-being.

The 2005 WHO *Bangkok Charter for Health Promotion in a Globalized World*[14] updated the definition to acknowledge the changes in commercialisation, globalisation, urbanisation and increasing inequalities since the *Ottawa Charter*:

Health promotion is the process of enabling people to increase control over their health and its determinants, and thereby improve their health. It is a core function of public health and contributes to the work of tackling communicable and non-communicable diseases and other threats to health.

Of particular relevance to OH nursing is the inclusion in the Bangkok Charter of a commitment to make the promotion of health a requirement of good corporate practices which may help to challenge the reluctance in some organisations to invest in health promotion.

Activity

It is worth looking at all these various definitions and from it writing your own based on your own experiences in practice. Discuss this with your colleagues or professional supervisor.

Having set the scene we will now move on to some of the theories underpinning health promotion activities, including health promotion models and behaviour change models; health needs assessment; and examples of workplace health promotion programmes.

Health promotion models

There are several different approaches to health promotion.

The medical approach

This is generally led by health professionals and focuses on the incidence and prevention of disease. A good example of the medical approach to health promotion is the immunisation programme in spring 2013 when an epidemic of measles spread through South Wales. It started in the Swansea area and was estimated to have affected nearly 1,000 people, including the death of a 25-year-old man. It then started to spread to the rest of the UK and plans were put in place to vaccinate over 1 million children to prevent further mortality. Although the medical approach is often criticised for not taking account of psychosocial factors it should not be discounted altogether. There is certainly benefit and value to be had from a medical approach programme such as immunisation, as evidenced by the eradication of smallpox.

The behavioural approach

This approach focuses on persuading people to make healthy changes to their lifestyle, although this does not necessarily address inequalities that may be affecting 'lifestyle choices'.

The educational approach

This assumes that providing sufficient information about health topics enables people to make informed choices about factors that affect their health. This can be problematic in the workplace as employers are keener on educating and training their employees to do the job and it takes a bit of convincing for them to see the benefits of lifestyle health promotion. OH nurses would also do well to remember the different educational, social and cultural backgrounds that employees come from.

The empowerment approach

The empowerment approach is based on the strategy outlined by the Ottawa Charter and is a long-term, community-based approach to empower people to gain control over their lives. However, it has been claimed that the workplace may not be the best place to use this approach.

The social change approach

This considers the broader socioeconomic and environmental perspectives. An example of this is the ban on smoking in public places which has been shown to be effective.[15]

Tannahill's model

Whilst it is not a specific approach to health promotion, Tannahill's model[9] is a useful way of understanding the topic (Figure 4.1). The three areas of health education, health protection and prevention all overlap and various OH nursing activities fall within the various spheres. For example, a hearing conservation programme may be considered as all three as it includes health protection (control of the hazard in the workplace), prevention (hearing surveillance) and health education (during the health surveillance medical). See Chapter 5 for more information on health surveillance.

Tannahill's model is widely accepted as a descriptive model of what happens in health promotion in OH. As can be seen in Figure 4.1, the model is based on three overlapping spheres. Examples of activities within these spheres would include:

- health education, e.g. health information on condition management given during a sickness absence review, such as information on how to manage low-back pain, healthy eating or the benefits of regular exercise
- health education/health protection, e.g. lobbying for a ban on tobacco advertising
- health protection, e.g. workplace smoking policy
- health protection/prevention, e.g. fluoride in drinking water
- prevention, e.g. risk assessment and the hierarchy of control to prevent risks to health in the workplace, giving immunisations where people are exposed to communicable diseases such as with healthcare workers
- prevention/health education, e.g. the education given to workers on hearing protection at their annual audiometry test
- all three spheres overlapping, e.g. a training segment on health in the induction training for new line managers.

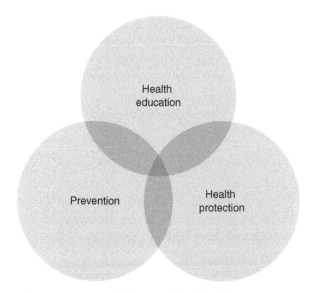

Figure 4.1 Tannahill's model of health promotion

Source: Tannahill (1985) cited by McFall T (2002) Health promotion and occupational health nursing. In: Oakley K (ed.) *Occupational Health Nursing*, 2nd edn. London: Whurr Publishers.

Other health promotion models

There is no comprehensive model for health promotion in the OH nursing sector but we can draw from existing models of health promotion.

Caplan and Holland (1990) used a four-paradigm model of health promotion based on the nature of society (from societal regulation to radical change) and the nature of knowledge (from subjective to objective).[16]

Beattie's (1991) model of health promotion places various health promotion activities within a four-part framework based on the mode of intervention (from authoritarian to negotiated) and the focus of intervention (from individual to collective), which may be more useful in the OH nursing setting.[17]

The French (1990)[18] model of health promotion seems more appropriate to primary care based as it is on disease management, health education, politics of health and disease prevention; whilst the Tones *et al.* (1990)[19] model is based on education and empowerment.

The Business in the Community Workwell model[20] considers health promotion in the business setting (Figure 4.2). The model is based on both employer and employee actions that should lead to clear business benefits. Employer actions include providing: a healthier physical and psychological environment; better work; better relationships; and better specialist support. Employee actions include being active; keeping learning; connecting with others; taking notice; and giving/volunteering. According to this model these actions work together to lead to greater productivity, improved engagement, better attendance, improved recruitment and retention and a better brand image.

Activity

Consider your own knowledge and experience and workplace setting in light of reading about these various health promotion models. Which models help you to underpin practice? Which models would you consider least helpful? How does the new Workwell model compare? Are there ways you can improve your own practice in promoting health after studying the models?

Behavioural change theories

Stages of change

Many health professionals will be familiar with the concept of stages of change.[8] It is one of the models used in smoking cessation and other health promotion activities and services. The idea is that behaviour change happens in stages:

1. precontemplation (not even considering behaviour change, such as quitting smoking)
2. contemplation (the person may recognise that behaviour change is necessary)

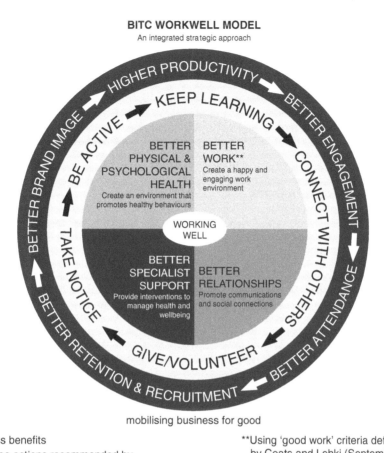

Figure 4.2 Business in the Community Workwell model

Source: Adapted from the BITC Workwell Model (2013). Available online at: http://www.bitc.org.uk/programmes/workwell/workwell-model.

3. preparation (preparing to make a behaviour change such as getting a prescription for nicotine replacement and setting a quit date)
4. action (actually making a change such as quitting smoking)
5. sustainment (maintaining the change such as remaining smokefree)
6. relapse (falling back to old habits such as restarting smoking, often after some type of stressor).

Stage-based psychological theories of change have been used by nurses in health promotion such as smoking cessation for some time. OH professionals who use brief interventions to promote health on an *ad hoc* basis will often seek to identify quickly which 'stage of change' the individual might be in with regard to their smoking in order to signpost appropriate services. For example, by identifying that an individual is thinking about trying to quit smoking (contemplation), giving the number of the local stop smoking service might be an effective intervention whereas it would not be effective if the individual was not interested in stopping smoking (precontemplation). Although this type of stages of change theory can be helpful when dealing with individuals by targeting the intervention at the individual's stage of change, it might not be so easily transferred to groups.

Continuum-based theories

Continuum-based psychological theories such as the health belief model aim to predict the variables involved in change and then focus on increasing or improving all those variables. Harrison *et al.*[21] described the health belief model in their meta-analysis of the use of the health belief model among adults in 1992. The health belief model was first developed in the 1960s and 1970s and is a value model which tries to explain individual health behaviour and behaviour change based on:

- the perception of the severity and likelihood of the health effect
- an evaluation of the behaviour change
- internal and external cues to action.

If we were to apply this theory to manual handling training we must consider the individuals' beliefs and perceptions about the risks from manual handling such as how likely they think it might be that they get injured and how severe they perceive the implications of injury to be. We should also address the individuals' evaluation of the behaviour change and empower them to see the benefits of making the change as outweighing the costs (e.g. the cost of giving up old ideas and ways of working). The intervention will also increase the external cues to action as the business attempts to change the culture through risk assessment and training. The Harrison *et al.* meta-analysis considered the four areas of susceptibility, severity, benefits and costs with regard to health behaviour. They concluded that further research was needed to understand how the four areas work together in order to validate the model.

In 2010 Carpenter[22] conducted a meta-analysis looking at the effectiveness of four variables within the health belief model in predicting behaviour (severity of negative health effect; individual susceptibility to the health effect; the benefits of the behaviour change in reducing likely outcome; perception of barriers to the behaviour) and found that benefits and barriers were the strongest predictors of behaviour. So by using a health belief model we can plan health promotion interventions so that we tackle the barriers to change and promote the benefits of behaviour change and tailor our health education, prevention and health protection activities.

Another exponent of the health belief models was DeJoy,[23] who applied a health belief model based on hazard appraisal, decision making, initiation and adherence to 'self-protective behaviour at work'. The principles of that model included threat-related beliefs (perception of severity and likelihood of negative health effect); self-efficacy (perceived ability to make the behaviour change); response efficacy (perceived effect of the behaviour change in reducing the risk of the negative health effect); and facilitating conditions and safety climate (benefits and costs of making the change). DeJoy suggested targeting the different areas to effect 'self-protective' behaviour change, taking account of the specific situation factors within the specific workplace.

Champion and Skinner[24] also outlined a comprehensive health belief model that includes modifying factors (age, gender, ethnicity, personality, knowledge, socioeconomics); personal/individual beliefs (perceived susceptibility and severity (threat), perceived benefits, perceived barriers and perceived self-efficacy); and actions (individual behaviours and cues to action). It has also been noted that research tends not to consider the effect of cues to action when evaluating the health belief model and so further research may be necessary to understand how these cues to action can be used to effect more positive change.[25]

One significant critique of health belief models is that they are based on cognitive processes and take no account of the emotional component of health beliefs and behaviour change.[24] For example, health beliefs about mammograms and cancer could be said to be particularly emotive and so focusing on cognitive health beliefs may not be enough to increase uptake of screening.

The role of the OH nurse

The first part of this chapter has demonstrated that health promotion is integral to the role of the OH nurse, as it is to any qualified nurse, whatever the discipline or area of practice.

The *Working for Health Equity: The role of health professionals* report[26] highlighted the very important responsibilities health professionals have in reducing health inequalities – responsibilities that have historically been underutilised. The report suggests various ways in which health professionals can tackle the social determinants of health to reduce health inequalities and promote health. The social determinants of health is a term used to describe the social and economic factors that can affect the overall health of a population, including factors affecting individual lifestyle choices. Examples include poverty and economic status; sanitation and housing; educational opportunities; and community cohesion. Thinking about these social factors can help us to design appropriate health promotion strategies. For example, a cooperative working together on an allotment growing fresh fruit and vegetables may provide some social support, self-esteem and community cohesion as well as affordable local food; it is suggested that this may have a bigger impact than a poster in a health centre telling people to eat more vegetables.

The Jakarta Declaration on leading health promotion into the twenty-first century[27] states that:

> The prerequisites for health are peace, shelter, education, social security, social relations, food, income, the empowerment of women, a stable eco-system, sustainable resource use, social justice, respect for human rights, and equity. Above all, poverty is the greatest threat to health.

It also cites demographic and other factors, including urbanisation, ageing society, increased sedentary behaviour, drug resistance, drug abuse, violence, new and re-emerging infectious diseases, and the need for greater recognition of mental health problems.

The *Working for Health Equity* report advocates education and training at undergraduate and postgraduate level for all health professionals to understand the social determinants of health. It also places importance on the need for health professionals to gather social history as well as medical history when making an assessment. It encourages health professionals to build relationships of trust with their clientele in order to tackle the social and economic factors affecting health so that they are able to signpost to other services where necessary. The aim here is to tackle the root causes of the problem as well as treating/medicating the health problem. The report also emphasises the role of health professionals as employers and managers and the need to utilise those roles to ensure staff health and wellbeing. Another key recommendation was partnership working both within and without the healthcare system with a focus on tackling the social determinants of health. They also recommend that individual health professionals and healthcare services act as advocates for individuals and groups and influence local and national policy to promote health. The statement for nurses, written by the Royal College of Nursing within the report, gives a set of principles that should underpin nursing practice in tackling inequalities. These include:

- all nurses, regardless of their work environment, knowing and understanding the health needs of their local population
- nurses identifying defined populations to enable healthcare teams to target individuals who would most benefit from preventive approaches
- nurses working in partnership with other members of health and social care organisations, to influence the work on tackling the wider determinants of health
- nurses engaging local people and groups, including those who are not in work, in public health awareness and action
- nurses making it their business to be informed, aware and responsive to disease outbreaks and other threats to health
- nurses utilising public health evidence in everyday practice, not just evidence for treating illness
- nurses working to public health knowledge and skills framework based on the 'novice to expert' criteria'.[25]

One role of the OH nurse in health promotion, and probably the one with they are most comfortable with, is as health educator. Nurses are often seen as being trustworthy sources of health information and have plenty of scope for sharing that information with individuals and groups.[28]

Another, maybe less comfortable, role in health promotion is that of role model for healthy lifestyles. Recent research[11] found that the majority of OH nurses felt that OH professionals should be role models in workplace health promotion. However, there was also wide consensus that they are often imperfect role models, a finding which was backed up by Rush *et al.*[29,30]

The OH nurse must work in partnership with others to deliver any kind of health service, including health promotion. Nurses are used to working with others in multidisciplinary teams, but in an occupational setting it is often necessary to work with lots of professionals outside healthcare. In a health promotion programme it may be necessary to work with human resources and health and safety colleagues as well as line managers, senior managers, employees and their representatives and various outside agencies. Some companies have found success by developing health promotion champions throughout the workforce to drive the health promotion programme and create healthy change. These champions rarely have any health background and in fact that is often the very reason that they work – health professionals in these types of programmes are seen as a resource rather than the drivers of the programme.

Much has been written about the importance of reform within nursing to allow us to fulfil our potential within health promotion and to move from our traditional role as health educators to tackling the wider scope of health promotion as part of a multiagency team.[7,31] This ties in with the author's own view that OH nurses have a vital role to play in improving the health and wellbeing of the working-age population but in order to do so they must become much less precious about protecting their area of expertise and embrace true multidisciplinary approaches.

Ethical considerations

The International Commission on OH gives the following ethical guidance:

> When engaging in health education, health promotion, health screening and public health programmes, OH professionals must seek the participation of both employers and workers in their design and in their implementation. They must also protect the confidentiality of personal health data of the workers, and prevent their misuse.[32]

The Nursing and Midwifery Council code of conduct[33] does not make specific reference to health promotion (or indeed to OH settings) but one of the main requirements of the code is for nurses to 'work with others to protect and promote the health and wellbeing of those in your care, their families and carers, and the wider community'.

Health promotion and the workplace setting

Although we have already highlighted the relevance of the workplace as a setting for health promotion it is important to understand the wider context. Health promotion is much wider than just tackling lifestyle issues and other factors will include socioeconomic status, job type, and health and social inequalities requiring multiagency and multilevel intervention. Likewise, health promotion initiatives can come from international, national, regional, local and organisational sources.[2,13,14,34]

Health needs analysis

Chapter 8 will cover OH needs assessment in more detail and will include an example of a general OH service needs assessment. The principles of needs analysis/assessment can also be applied to health promotion. It is important to involve all the stakeholders in identifying and prioritising topics for health promotion as the topics that may seem important to the individual OH nurse may not be important to the employer or to the employees, leading to a waste of resources whilst the important issues are not dealt with and opportunities for real improvement in health and wellbeing are missed. Once the topics have been identified and prioritised it is still important to have input from a variety of people in order for health promotion activities to be appropriate. Language can be as important as the message and this is an area in which medical professionals, including nurses, can fall foul; a message that makes sense to us may not mean the same thing to the audience for which it is intended. This may be due to regional differences, jargon, generational differences or various other causes. The medium of delivery may also need thought. A photocopied leaflet may have all the relevant information but it may be received better if delivered by interactive email or social media.

A health needs analysis or assessment is a sensible thing to do before considering any specific health promotion activities. A systematic approach to reviewing the health status and health needs of the organisation will improve the effectiveness of any health promotion activity as well as increasing cost benefit to the organisation, which is particularly important during times of economic pressure.

A needs assessment should demonstrate clear, measurable benefits for the chosen initiatives as well as setting the indicators for evaluating the effectiveness of the service or initiative. It involves all stakeholders (senior management, line managers, employees, unions, human resources, health and safety, OH) and although it does not need to be led by OH, they should certainly be involved.

Interventions should be targeted based on the outcome of the health needs assessment and should be delivered in a variety of ways to maximise access, convenience, fun, engagement and freshness.[35]

The National Institute for Health and Clinical Excellence (NICE) defined health needs assessment as 'a systematic method for reviewing the health issues facing a population leading to agreed priorities and resource allocation that will improve health and reduce inequalities'. They have produced a useful document describing how to conduct a health needs assessment which includes case studies from various settings, including workplaces.

The NICE guidance suggests a five-step approach to health needs assessment:

1. getting started
2. identifying health priorities
3. assessing a health priority for action
4. action planning for change
5. moving on/project review.

The guidance is clear. Although the process is presented in a linear fashion, in practice it is usually necessary to revisit various points several times and so it is worth being aware of the whole process from the outset.

Once the team of stakeholders has been identified then it is necessary to assemble information which may include risk assessments, sickness absence records, OH referrals, management or union concerns and records of claims. There should then be a discussion of health issues with all levels in the organisation through focus groups or surveys. Consideration should also be given to the specific workplace population to ensure that interventions will be suitable. Likewise, consideration should be given to both the effects of work on health, e.g. ergonomics, noise, chemicals, stress, as well as the effects of health on work, e.g. obesity, smoking, alcohol and drug use.

Once the health promotion issues in your organisation have been identified by the health needs assessment it is then necessary to plan the intervention. This planning should be guided by the questions:

- Where are you going?
- How will you get there?
- What do you need to be able to do that?
- When you get there, has it been successful?

Defining the initiative and its objectives at the outset will help to ensure that all stakeholders are in agreement and support the initiative. The group should decide how that will be done and what resources are needed for the project. A group approach to this will help to identify factors that may otherwise be overlooked. For example, introducing fresh food to vending machines may require increased visits to stock, clean and refill the vending machines and possibly increased waste if food has to be discarded. Smoking cessation groups will require space and time but may also need printed information, a carbon monoxide monitor and nicotine replacement therapies. Although a smoking cessation group held after working hours might reduce the cost of staff time it might increase other costs such as heat and light.

Objectives should be SMART:

- specific
- measurable
- achievable
- realistic
- time-bound.

Evaluation of health promotion initiatives is often overlooked. However, the approach above will set out the parameters against which the initiative can be evaluated. Although cost benefit is often given priority, it may not always be the best measure for these initiatives, whilst measures such as pounds in weight loss, cigarettes saved or sickness absence improved may be better.

See case studies 4.1–4.3 for examples of health promotion programmes in OH.

Case study 4.1   Manual handling

Smith and Son is a medium-sized company in the south of England which manufactures medical equipment. They engaged the services of an occupational health and safety company after receiving an improvement notice from the Health and Safety Executive (HSE) for manual handling. The initial assessment therefore focused on manual handling as the main, most urgent topic for health promotion. After consultation with human resources, senior management, line management, the IT department and employee representatives, a training programme was designed as a workplace health promotion intervention. This training programme was in two parts, with an e-learning module written by an OH specialist and a practical, on-site session led by an OH nurse. The e-learning module covered the risk of injury from manual handling, the use of manual handling aids and the principles of safe manual handling and introduced the acronym TILE (task, individual, load and environment) for use in assessing manual handling tasks.

The practical sessions involved up to 15 employees from different departments, including manufacturing, production, logistics, service, maintenance, welding, sales and field service. The session started with a review of TILE and other aspects of the e-learning before going into the workplace to look at specific manual handling tasks. Mixing up groups of employees helped them to see other roles and tasks within the company which helped with their sense of teamwork. It also helped to have 'fresh eyes' looking at regular tasks within individuals' daily work and identifying unsafe practice and better solutions to manual handling problems. The manual handling training was one part of a programme of improvement which included reviewing risk assessments, reorganising stock areas to clear out unused tooling and other goods, changing processes to make use of trolleys and reorganising shelves, taking the weight of stock items into account. Evaluation of the programme included feedback from employees, return inspection by HSE and reduced accidents or incidents related to manual handling.

Source: Edwards S (2012) Handle with care. *Occup Hlth* (July). Available online at: http://www.personneltoday.com/articles/01/10/2012/58636/cutting-health-risks-through-manual-handling-training.htm#.UYALY8rpzvh.

Case study 4.2   Lifestyle

GlaxoSmithKline

GlaxoSmithKline[36] have introduced global programmes of health promotion to all their employees, including in countries with expensive or inadequate healthcare systems. Their Energy for Performance and Personal Resilience (E4P) programme is a well-established training programme that aims to help employees reduce stress in the workplace and at home and increase energy and productivity levels. The course includes nutrition, exercise and rest and the company has 'energy champions' to coach and support employees in the workplace after they have been through the training programme. The newer programme, called Partnership for Prevention, is a bigger commitment that offers a range of health promotion and prevention services, including smoking cessation, cancer screening, HIV screening and treatment and immunisations to all employees and their dependants.

Ginsters

Ginsters[37] (the pasty people) found that the majority of their employees did not take regular exercise and were therefore at greater risk of health problems as a result. Ginsters developed a programme called Active Workplace, in partnership with their local council and Sport England. The programme includes health assessments and advice, including weight loss, exercise and smoking cessation; access to a free gym on site 24 hours a day; free taster sessions for up to 80 different activities, including surfing, canoeing and archery; and subsidised activities for employees and their families. On evaluation of the programme Ginsters found that in excess of 80 per cent of their employees had taken up some of these activities and made a more active lifestyle a reality.

Food and Drink Federation

The Food and Drink Federation have published details of several workplace wellbeing schemes in large companies in the UK and you can read more about them at http://www.fdf.org.uk/publicgeneral/FINALFDFWorkplaceWellbeingBrochure.pdf.

Case study 4.3   Cardiac health

Hampton Knight – partnership working with the NHS public health teams

Hampton Knight are providers of occupational health (OH) services. Working with their client, a leading global engineering company, and the NHS, Hampton Knight provided targeted educational support to employees around the benefits of improving cardiac health.

In 2012, following two cardiac arrests on the client site, a number of serious cardiac medical emergencies and increasing 'cardiac-related' sickness absence

(continued)

(continued)

within one of the assembly lines, Hampton Knight approached the organisation to undertake a proactive pilot study to identify potential health issues.

With support from management, human resources (HR) and the union, and working collaboratively with the NHS Healthy Living Team, 122 employees attended a Lifestyle Health Event. Participants were asked to complete a lifestyle questionnaire and underwent a series of physical health measurements.

Demonstrating a corporate responsibility and commitment to improving health and wellbeing, employees were given time to attend the event, away from production, which did not encroach on their free time or breaks.

The results

The pilot study looked at 100 randomly selected lifestyle questionnaires and physical health measurements, consisting of body mass index (BMI), waist measurements, blood pressure and carbon monoxide monitoring for smokers. Participants, randomly selected, were all male. However, to put this into context, only one participant out of the 122 people surveyed was female. This pilot study sample group is reflective of the site demographics, as employees within manufacturing are predominantly male.

Statistically significant findings from the pilot study revealed:

- an ageing workforce – 77 per cent of employees were aged between 37 and 64 years
- 88 per cent work shifts including nightshift
- large 'at-risk' group for developing high blood pressure – 39 per cent
- 61 per cent of the study were overweight
- 18 per cent of the study participants were obese (BMI over 30)
- 26 per cent of the study took no exercise
- 80 per cent of the study did not eat 'five a day'
- employee perception is that 'work is enough' exercise, therefore they did no additional exercise away from work
- 74 per cent were non-smokers
- 94 per cent consumed less than 21 units of alcohol per week.

Feedback of results to employees

In order to address these issues, OH and the NHS Healthy Living Team organised an event to feed back the results and provide educational support around the benefits of maintaining a healthy lifestyle. The event was widely publicised to increase attendance. Support from the local branch of a global supermarket chain was gained; free leaflets and fruit were donated and given out on the day.

Nutritional advice

Employees were given the opportunity to speak to a member of the on-site catering department to advise on guideline daily amounts for products available to purchase on site. The concept of 'healthy lunch boxes' was introduced, along with the benefits of eating healthily and its link to improvements in physical health and mental wellbeing.

Smoking cessation

The NHS Healthy Living Team attended the feedback event. One-to-one smoking cessation advice was given and referrals to Stop Smoking clinics were available on the day.

Personal trainer

Although the assembly line requires some physical work, this is limited to upper-body movement and is not deemed to be cardiovascularly challenging. An opportunity to access a free personal trainer on site for 10 weeks was offered to employees. The one-to-one sessions were specific to the needs of each individual, taking into consideration lifestyle factors, health problems and personal goals.

Free gym passes

Supported by a local gym, free one-day passes for gym membership were issued to those seeking to increase their exercise.

Team challenge

The OH team challenged groups of four employees to walk the distance equal to from Land's End to John O'Groats over 4 weeks, by means of a 10,000 steps a day pedometer challenge. Following keen interest from other areas within the factory, the intention is to introduce a larger-scale challenge across the site over the summer period. Working in collaboration with the local Championship football team and Premiership rugby team, prizes were keenly donated, to help incentivise participation.

The study challenged preconceived opinions that the incidence of smoking and alcohol would be high amongst these factory workers. It revealed that in reality diet and exercise were the two key problem areas and from this a targeted health promotion initiative was developed and implemented. The results provided visible and valuable data to demonstrate to workers, management, union and HR employees' risk of developing cardiac ill health due to a combination of issues, including shift work, poor diet and lack of exercise.

(continued)

(continued)

The future: work4wellness

The OH department launched work4wellness, a 3-year targeted health promotion strategy prompted by this study. The goal is to provide employees with opportunities whilst at work to develop healthier habits, attitudes and behaviours, which will positively contribute to improved physical health and mental wellbeing.

The work4wellness logo is now present on all health promotion material visible across the site. Health promotion interventions include monthly toolbox talks on varying health topics; an OH newsletter and website; quarterly wellness events in line with national initiatives; and an annual Health Fayre. The theme of the 2013 Health Fayre focuses on preventing cardiac ill health and promoting wellbeing. The event is open to all; national charities and organisations are invited to attend and employees are provided with the opportunity to talk to specialists in their field and gain further insight into a variety of major health problems.

Building upon the positive journey so far, the OH team will continue to strive towards fostering working relationships with the NHS, national charities, local organisations and professional sports teams, with the aim of developing a healthy workforce characterised by staff who understand what they can do as individuals to maintain their own health and actively pursue this.

Hampton Knight OH team comprises Julie Routledge, OH Manager, Vicky Edwards and Claire Izod.

Evaluation

The nursing process is a basic building block for nursing practice, including OH nursing. It is a problem-solving approach and was first introduced into nursing in the USA in the 1950s and in the UK in the 1970s,[38] although it has developed since then. The stages of the nursing process are:

1. assess
2. (diagnose – this step was added later)
3. plan
4. implement
5. evaluate.

Evaluation, the last step, is as important as any of the other steps in the process but unfortunately is often forgotten or dismissed as not necessary. When designing any health promotion initiatives it is as important to plan for evaluation as it is for the other stages. The criteria for evaluation should be agreed at the outset and may need to be wider than a simple return on investment calculation. For example, a stop smoking initiative may want to consider number of cigarettes saved or weeks of smoking cessation achieved as well as considering the cost of the initiative. Likewise, a weight loss initiative may consider pounds or inches lost in the evaluation alongside sickness absence levels. It is also important to remember that the nursing process is cyclical rather than linear. Evaluation should inform the ongoing process and any future health promotion initiatives on the topic, not just be a bookend to complete the activity.

Costs for health promotion should be both planned for and evaluated. One obvious cost is the time needed for the people to undertake the whole exercise, including the planning, implementation and evaluation of the activity. Other costs will need to be taken into account, for example, in a healthy eating initiative the possible increase in costs to clean and stock vending machines with fresh produce and the possible increase in waste with shorter use-by dates.

Naidoo and Wills[8] use a handy 5E mnemonic for evaluation:

1. effort
2. efficiency
3. effectiveness
4. execution
5. efficacy.

So evaluation should consider what resources have been used (effort) and whether that was an economically sound use of resources (efficiency), measure the impact of the programme and whether it achieved its outcomes (effectiveness), evaluate the appropriateness of the method employed (execution) and assess the overall benefit of the intervention (efficacy). Evaluation should then inform future programmes.

Tones[39] discusses some of the pitfalls of evaluating health promotion initiatives, particularly when approached from a medical perspective with its reliance on random control trials as the only valid way of assessing evidence. He outlines some examples of potentially 'successful' interventions that may be classed as 'failures' or not effective by incorrect evaluation techniques. So, for example, a particular intervention may be very effective for a certain group within the main population but not make any difference to other groups: if the intervention is evaluated on its effect on the whole population, its success may be watered down.

Activity

Consider any health promotion you have undertaken in your practice. How did you evaluate it? What did you do with the evaluation? Did it inform any further health promotion activities and if so, how? In light of what you have read, what changes would you make to any health promotion programmes in your workplace?

Conclusion

This chapter has laid out the argument that health promotion is a key aspect of OH nursing. Although nurses have traditionally been trusted as health educators, it has already been acknowledged that health promotion is much wider than that and includes the spheres of prevention, health protection and health education. There are also social determinants of health and health inequalities that the OH nurse must be aware of and consider with any health promotion project. It is essential that, in order to fulfil their vital role in health promotion, OH nurses work in partnership and cooperation with other stakeholders if they are to improve the health and wellbeing of the population with which they are working.

References

1 International Council of Nursing (12.04.2010) *Nursing Definition*. Available online at: http://www.icn.ch/about-icn/icn-definition-of-nursing (accessed 16.10.12).
2 Whitaker S, Baranski B (2001) *The Role of the Occupational Health Nurse in Workplace Health Management*. Copenhagen: World Health Organization. Available online at: http://www.who.int/occupational_health/regions/en/oeheurnursing.pdf.
3 Bagley D (2002) The role of the occupational health nurse. In: Oakley K (ed.) *Occupational Health Nursing*, 2nd edn. London: Whurr Publishers.
4 Thornbory G (2009) What is occupational health? In: Thornbory G (ed.) *Public Health Nursing: A textbook for health visitors, school nurses and occupational health nurses*. Chichester: Wiley-Blackwell.
5 Hutchinson AD, Wilson C (2011) Improving nutrition and physical activity in the work-place: A meta-analysis of intervention studies. *Hlth Promotion Int* 27(2): 238–249.
6 http://www.who.int/about/definition/en/print.html.
7 Noblet AJ, Rodwell JJ (2010) Workplace health promotion. In: Leva S, Houdmont J *Occupational Health Psychology*. Chichester: Wiley-Blackwell.
8 Naidoo J, Wills J (2009) *Foundations for Health Promotion,* 3rd edn. Edinburgh: Baillière-Tindall.
9 Tannahill A (1985) cited by McFall T (2002) Health promotion and occupational health nursing. In: Oakley K (ed.) *Occupational Health Nursing,* 2nd edn. London: Whurr Publishers.
10 Naidoo J, Wills J (2010) *Developing Practice for Public Health and Health Promotion,* 3rd edn. Edinburgh: Baillière-Tindall.
11 Edwards S (2012) Should occupational health professionals be role models in workplace health promotion? MSc dissertation, unpublished.
12 US Department of Health and Human Services (2005) *Theory at a Glance: A guide for health promotion practice,* 2nd edn. Available online at: http://www.cancer.gov/cancertopics/cancerlibrary/theory.pdf.
13 World Health Organization (1986) *Ottawa Charter.* Available online at: http://www.who.int/healthpromotion/conferences/previous/ottawa/en/index.html.
14 WHO (2005) *Bangkok Charter for Health Promotion in a Globalized World.* Available online at: http://www.who.int/healthpromotion/conferences/6gchp/hpr_050829_%20BCHP.pdf.
15 http://www.smokefreeengland.co.uk/files/dhs01_01-one-year-on-report-final.pdf.

16 Caplan R, Holland R (1990) Rethinking health education theory. *Health Educ J* 49: 1.

17 Beattie A (1991) Knowledge and control in health promotion: A test case for social policy and theory. In: Gabe J, Calnan M, Bury M (eds) *The Sociology of the Health Service*. London: Routledge.

18 French J (1990) Boundaries and horizons, the role of health education within health promotion. *Health Educ J* 49: 1.

19 Tones K, Tilford S, Robinson Y (1990) *Health Education: Effectiveness and efficiency*. London: Chapman and Hall.

20 BITC Workwell Model (2013) Available online at: http://www.bitc.org.uk/programmes/workwell/workwell-model.

21 Harrison JA, Mullen PD, Green LW (1992) A meta-analysis of studies of the health belief model with adults. *Health Educ Res* 7 (1): 107–116.

22 Carpenter CJ (2010) A meta-analysis of the effectiveness of health belief model variables in predicting behaviour. *Health Commun* 25 (8): 661–669.

23 DeJoy DM (1996) Theoretical models of health behaviour and workplace: Self-protective behaviour. *J Saf Res* 27: 61–72.

24 Champion VL, Skinner CS (2008) The health belief model. In: Glanz K, Rimer BK, Viswanath K (eds) *Health Behaviour and Health Education: Theory, research and practice*, 4th edn. San Francisco, CA: John Wiley.

25 Rimer K (2008) Models of individual health behaviour. In: Glanz K, Rimer BK, Viswanath K (eds) *Health Behaviour and Health Education: Theory, research and practice*, 4th edn. San Francisco, CA: John Wiley.

26 UCL Institute for Health Equity (2013) *Working for Health Equity: The role of health professionals*. London: UCL. Available online at: http://www.instituteofhealthequity.org.

27 WHO (1997) *The Jakarta Declaration on Leading Health Promotion into the 21st Century*. Available online at: http://www.who.int/healthpromotion/Milestones_Health_Promotion_05022010.pdf.

28 Clarke A (1991) Nurses as role models and health educators. *J Adv Nurs* 16: 1178–1184.

29 Rush KL, Kee CC, Rice M (2010) The self as role model in health promotion scale: Development and testing. *West J Nurs Res* 32(6): 814–832. Available online at: http://wjn.sagepub.com/content/32/6/814.

30 Rush KL, Kee CC, Rice M (2005) Nurses as imperfect role models for health promotion. *West J NursiRes* 27(2): 166–183. Available online at: http://wjn.sagepub.com/content/27/2/166.

31 Whitehead D (2009) Reconciling the differences between health promotion in nursing and 'general' health promotion. *Int J Nurs Studies* 46: 865–874.

32 International Commission on Occupational Health (2012) *Code of Ethics*. Available online at: http://www.icohweb.org/site_new/multimedia/core_documents/pdf/code_ethics_eng_2012.pdf.

33 Nursing and Midwifery Council (2008) *The Code: Standards of conduct, performance and ethics for nurses and midwives*. Available online at: http://www.nmc-uk.org/Documents/Standards/The-code-A4-20100406.pdf.

34 *NICE Guidance Guides Related to OH*. Available online at: http://www.nice.org.uk/guidance/index.jsp?action=bypublichealth&PUBLICHEALTH=Occupational+health#/search/?reload.

35 National Institute for Health and Clinical Excellence (2009) *Health Needs Assessment: A practical guide*. Available online at: http://www.nice.org.uk/media/150/35/Health_Needs_Assessment_A_Practical_Guide.pdf.

36 *GlaxoSmithKline Annual Report* (2012) Available online at: http://www.gsk.com/content/dam/gsk/globals/documents/pdf/corporateresponsibility/cr-report-2012/gsk-cr-2012-report.pdf.

37 http://www.ginsters.co.uk/social-responsibility/ginsters-active-workplace-scheme.

38 Hincliff S, Norman S, Schober J (1998) *Nursing Practice and Health Care: A foundation text,* 3rd edn. London: Arnold.

39 Tones K (2000) Evaluating health promotion: A tale of three errors. *Patient Educ Counselling* 39: 227–236. Available online at: http://www.uic.edu/sph/prepare/courses/chsc433/tones.pdf.

5 Health surveillance

Susanna Everton

Learning objectives

After reading this chapter you will be able to:

- appreciate what health surveillance is and what it is not
- discuss the legal, ethical and financial reasons for health surveillance
- discuss hazard identification, risk assessment and workplace inspection
- explore the role of occupational health (OH) professionals in health surveillance
- appreciate what records and record management are required for health surveillance
- appreciate how to work as part of the OH and safety team
- describe the principles of prevention and appreciate where personal protective equipment (PPE) fits with health surveillance.

What is health surveillance?

OH surveillance is about systematically watching for early signs of work-related ill health in employees exposed to certain health risks. It means putting in place procedures to achieve this. The employer or designated person will have identified those activities hazardous to health, the employees at risk and the measures taken to eliminate or reduce the risks. The International Labour Organization[1] (p. 22) defined OH surveillance as:

> the on-going systematic collection, analysis, interpretation and dissemination of data for the purpose of prevention. Surveillance is essential to the planning, implementation and evaluation of OH programmes and to the control of work-related ill health and injuries, as well as to the protection and promotion of workers' health. OH surveillance includes workers' health surveillance and working environment surveillance.

OH surveillance must not be confused with general screening, e.g. tests and health assessments, both physical and psychological, performed on employees as part of their general fitness or fitness to work. These may include health assessment for night workers, pregnant women and those returning to work after childbirth, as well as medicals for drivers, divers and heavy goods vehicle licence holders. There has to be a connection between the health risk, the activity and the management of preventive controls.

OH surveillance usually takes the form of a periodic clinical screening and/or medical examination of individuals who may be exposed to harmful substances or physical hazards which may affect their health. The tests need to be standardised and reproducible, which in practice can exclude those where a subjective assessment is the only test available. OH surveillance is therefore often limited to tests and examination for hearing loss, lung function, skin disorders and blood tests for lead levels. The OH individual responsible for the programme should have a written health surveillance procedure which is also available to the employer, individual, safety team and staff representatives so that all are aware of what is to be done, by whom and what happens to the information. This should include:

- identification of the health hazard and risk
- identification of the exposed group
- setting an allocated period for the targeted health screening
- details of the health examination required:

  o   health questionnaire
  o   test or procedure
  o   medical examination if required

- discussion of results with individual referral if required
- use and management of records, including the health record
- report to management on individual and group
- arrangement for continuing surveillance.

The purposes of health surveillance can be described as a way of detecting any special vulnerability to particular hazards and establishing a baseline health status from which to monitor change which will also require an awareness of those with pre-existing health problems. It is also available to:

- identify any changes to health from an early stage to allow for intervention and instigate remedial measures
- comply with statutory requirements for specific occupations or hazards[2]
- check the effectiveness of control measures in the risk assessment
- inform management, employees and their representatives to enhance risk management.

As a way of measuring the effectiveness of the control, targeted groups of workers can be checked providing there are validated and standardised tests available. These can be at three levels:

1. simple visual examination, e.g. for skin disorders
2. specific technical tests, e.g. hearing tests for those exposed to noise, lung functions for those exposed to dusts or allergens

3. medical examination and tests, e.g. for upper-limb disorders, blood tests for lead levels, X-ray for lung disorders.

Results from these groups can be presented as anonymised data to managers as well as highlighting individuals who may be particularly at risk, thus informing the managers on whether their control measures are effective, or which workers may be particularly at risk.

Legal requirements

Health surveillance is required by law for some hazards, under the Management of Health and Safety at Work Regulations 1999:[3]

> **6** Every employer shall ensure that his employees are provided with such health surveillance as is appropriate having regard to the risks to their health and safety which are identified by the assessment.

This is further supported by legislation in the Control of Substances Hazardous to Health Regulations 1999 (2002)[4] (COSHH):

> **11 (1)** Where it is appropriate for the protection of the health of his employees who are, or are liable to be exposed to a substance hazardous to health, the employer shall ensure that such employees are under suitable health surveillance.

These cover most work situations except where the following Regulations apply:

- 5 (1) (i) The Coal Mines (Control of Inhalable Dust) Regulations 2007[5]
- (ii) The Control of Lead at Work Regulations 2002[6]
- (iii) The Control of Asbestos at Work Regulations 2002.[7]

Other legislation where there is a requirement for health surveillance:

- The Control of Noise at Work Regulations 2005[8]
- The Control of Vibration at Work Regulations 2005[9]
- The Ionising Radiation at Work Regulations 1999.[10]

The law requires the employee, to whom health or medical surveillance applies, to present him- or herself during working hours and at the employer's expense, for any surveillance procedures and provide any relevant health information requested.

Under the requirements of Chemical Hazards Information and Packaging Regulations 2009 (CHIP4),[11] all hazardous substances must be clearly labelled with relevant safety, health and environmental information. Take a look at products and containers used in the workplace, and you will see the labels, pictograms and information (Figure 5.1). Online management systems for COSHH assessments are now available to assist employers in managing their particular risks. REACH is a new European Union regulation concerning the registration, evaluation, authorisation and restriction of chemicals.[12] It came into force on 1 June 2007 and replaces a number of European Directives and Regulations with a single system, and is the legal authority for hazard data sheets.

	Acute toxicity – oral, dermal, inhalation Categories 1, 2, 3
	Skin corrosion categories 1A, 1B, 1C Serious eye damage category 1

	Acute toxicity – oral, dermal, inhalation category 4
	Skin irritation categories 2, 3
	Eye irritation category 2A
	Skin sensitisation category 1
	Specific target organ toxicity following single exposure category 3
	    Respiratory tract irritation
	    Narcotic effects

	Respiratory sensitisation category 1 Germ cell mutagenicity category 1A, 1B, 2 Carcinogenicity category 1A, 1B, 2 Reproductive toxicity category 1A, 1B, 2 Specific target organ toxicity following single exposure category 1, 2 Specific target organ toxicity following repeated exposure category 1, 2 Aspiration hazard category 1, 2
No image	Acute toxicity – oral, dermal, inhalation category 5 Eye irritation category 2B Reproductive toxicity – effects on or via lactation

Figure 5.1 New pictograms to meet international standards

Ethical requirements

In setting up a health surveillance programme in the workplace, it is not enough just to consider employees' exposure and the tests that can be carried out. There is an ethical responsibility for the personal information that is collected, on how that information is used and how it is stored – see Data Protection Act 1998.[13] There is also an ethical requirement to ensure that any tests or examinations are actually necessary and can be justified. The International Labour Organization published guidelines in 1998[1] (p. v) which are still relevant today, offering assistance 'to all those who have responsibilities to design, establish, implement and manage workers' health surveillance schemes that

Workers' health surveillance, within an organized framework, should be based on sound ethical and technical practice. Specifically, any workers' health surveillance programme must ensure:

(i) professional independence and impartiality of the relevant health professionals;
(ii) workers' privacy and confidentiality of individual health information.

Procedures in a particular programme must meet, clearly and demonstrably, four criteria of worth or value: need, relevance, scientific validity and effectiveness.

2.6. The collection, analysis and communication of workers' health information should lead to action. The particular programme must relate the results of the programme to its declared purposes, and must identify what the consequences will be for workers' health and livelihood (work, job security/income), and what the impact of the programme will be on the structure of the workplace and working conditions.

6.12. The employer, in consultation with workers' representatives and the joint safety and health committees, where they exist, may offer medical surveillance and health promotion programmes to workers in their employment, preferably within the framework of organized occupational health services.

6.13. The employer may request from occupational health professionals anonymous, collective health-related information for prevention purposes and should be given appropriate and relevant information for taking effective measures to protect workers' health and to prevent further occurrences of occupational accidents and health disorders.

6.14. If a particular job is found medically contra-indicated for a worker, the employer must make every effort to find alternative employment or another appropriate solution, such as retraining or facilitating access to social benefits, rehabilitation or a pension scheme.

Figure 5.2 Key points for a health surveillance programme

Source: International Labour Organization (1998) *Technical and Ethical Guidelines for Workers' Health Surveillance*. Geneva: International Labour Organization, pp. 2, 15.

will facilitate preventative actions towards ensuring a healthy and safe working environment for all'. A summary of the main points can be found in Figure 5.2.

Ethical dilemmas can also occur when considering exposing employees to known hazards which may be essential to an industrial process. But what is an acceptable risk? The fundamental concept of acceptable risk is subjective and is determined by various courses of actions that have different levels of consequence. Fischhoff *et al.*[14] (p. 3) state that:

One does not accept risks, one accepts options that entail some level of risk among their consequence. Whenever the decision-making process has taken into account benefits or other (no-risk) costs, the most acceptable option need not be the one with the least risk . . . one might choose (or accept) the option with the highest risk if it had enough compensating benefits.

The World Health Organization[15] issued a list of standpoints for determining when risk is acceptable (for water quality), some of which are relevant in OH and safety. A risk is acceptable when:

- it falls below an arbitrary defined probability
- it falls below some level that is already tolerated

- it falls below an arbitrary defined attributable fraction of total disease burden in the community
- the cost of reducing the risk would exceed the costs saved
- the cost of reducing the risk would exceed the costs saved when the 'costs of suffering' are also factored in
- the opportunity costs would be better spent on other, more pressing, public health problems
- public health professionals say it is acceptable
- the general public say it is acceptable (or more likely, do not say it is not)
- politicians say it is acceptable.

Confidentiality

Confidentiality is another area which causes ethical problems. The person who is running the health surveillance programme has a responsibility to the employer and to the employee as well as to his or her own professional body and codes of conduct and colleagues. This can often cause a conflict of interest[16] so it is appropriate to be aware of ethical codes on confidentiality and medical reports that are available from the Faculty of Occupational Medicine, and the codes of professional conduct for nurses and midwives from the Nursing and Midwifery Council.

Information on the health of an employee given to a healthcare professional, such as a doctor or nurse, can only be passed on to a third party in exceptional circumstances (see section on Confidentiality in Chapter 1), or only with the informed consent of the individual. In a health surveillance context if details of a medical nature are disclosed to the OH practitioner, then these must be kept separate from the health record as they are confidential. The legal position on confidentiality in OH is discussed by Lewis and Thornbory,[17] Kloss[18] and Kloss and Ballard.[19]

Financial requirements

Sickness absence costs

According to analysis of sickness absence, most sickness absence is not caused or made worse by the workplace.[20] Statistics quoted by Black[20] suggest that only around one-fifth of working days lost to sickness absence are work-related (around 22 million days due to work-related ill health and a further 4.4 million to workplace injury). However the cost to the individual, the organisation and society in general for ill health at work is often not measurable.

Benefit costs

Certain listed illnesses fall into the category eligible for compensation via Industrial Injuries Disablement Benefit (IIDB) (Figure 5.3). Claims for IIDB should be made to

Claims for **Industrial Injuries Disablement Benefit** can be made if the employee was employed in a job that caused his or her disease. The scheme covers more than 70 diseases, including:

- Asthma
- Chronic bronchitis or emphysema
- Sensorineural hearing loss
- Pneumoconiosis (including silicosis and asbestosis)
- Osteoarthritis of the knee in coal miners
- Prescribed disease A11 (previously known as vibration white finger)
- Peripheral neuropathy

The scheme also covers asbestos-related diseases, including:

- Pneumoconiosis (asbestosis)
- Diffuse mesothelioma
- Primary carcinoma of the lung with asbestosis
- Primary carcinoma of the lung without asbestosis but where there has been extensive occupational exposure to asbestos in specified occupations
- Unilateral or bilateral pleural thickening

Figure 5.3 Conditions for claims via Industrial Injuries Disablement Benefit

Source: https://www.gov.uk/industrial-injuries-disablement-benefit/overview.

the Department for Work and Pensions. This industrial injuries compensation is paid by the taxpayer, not by the employer, and is no-fault; that is, it is not necessary to prove negligence. However, if the employer is at fault the worker may have a separate and additional claim for compensation through the civil law of tort. Such claims, if successful, may lead to increased insurance premiums and bad publicity for the company, especially if the case is high-profile or involved a large number of employees. The Ministry of Justice[21] has produced a protocol for those seeking to make a personal injury claim where the injury is not the result of an accident at work but takes the form of an illness or disease. A few cases are prosecuted in the criminal courts under health and safety legislation, and may lead to criminal convictions and fines, or even exceptionally a term of imprisonment for senior managers.

Those who believe their ill health was as a result of work or a work exposure will also need to have that diagnosed by an appropriate occupational physician and reported under the Reporting of Injuries, Diseases and Dangerous Occurrences Regulations 1995 (RIDDOR)[22] (currently undergoing review). These compensations are paid by the taxpayer – where is the penalty for the employer who was responsible for the illness or injury? This may be apparent in higher company insurance, loss of reputation, particularly if a large number of employees have been involved, the case has hit the media or the employee has made a claim. Some cases go to court under health and safety legislation and the employer can be penalised through fines or occasionally criminal convictions.

As it is a statutory requirement to manage health risks in the workplace, then the cost of a basic health surveillance where it is required will be a good business case for most employers, and the actual costs of implementing a programme can be managed if a systematic approach is made.

Hazard identification and risk assessment

The Management of Health and Safety at Work Regulations 1999[3] place an absolute duty on employers to undertake a risk assessment of:

- the risks to the health and safety of their employees to which they are exposed whilst they are at work
- the risks to the health and safety of persons not in their employment arising out of or in connection with the conduct by them of their undertakings.

When discussing risk assessment it is important not to confuse terms. The assessment is looking at the *hazard* – the activity employees are undertaking or the substances they may be using that could cause them ill health or injury and the likelihood of that outcome occurring – the *risk*. To ease understanding, a hazard can be defined as a substance or agent which possesses the potential of producing harm. Hazards can therefore be physical, chemical, biological or psychological. A risk depends upon the probability of harm being produced. An estimate of the degree of risk is possible if there is a measure of both hazard and exposure to employees. See Figure 5.4 for an example of a risk matrix.

The OH nurse adviser and team should know the business of the organisation employing them to run the health surveillance programme. They should know what the employees do, where they do it and what they might be exposed to; they should talk with the managers, the employees and the safety team and undertake informal or formal inspections of the workplace. Understanding what could cause harm to health puts the OH adviser in a better position to advise on what may be done to control the risk.

The risk assessment should be carried out by a competent individual – someone with experience and knowledge of the activity or substance and with the ability to devise practical controls that can be implemented, and reviewed effectively. This responsibility usually falls on the manager of the relevant area who can be assisted by safety advisers and specialists. Where health surveillance is statutorily required or identified as part of the controls, then an OH adviser should be consulted. Some hazards may require medical surveillance, in which case an appropriately qualified medical practitioner will be engaged. Sometimes it works the other way around – the OH adviser will recognise a health problem for a particular area from routine health screening or from

Potential severity of harm	Likelihood of harm occurring		
	1 = Unlikely	2 = Likely	3 = Highly likely
1 = Slightly harmful	1 = Trivial	2 = Tolerable	3 = Moderate
2 = Harmful	2 = Tolerable	4 = Moderate	6 = Substantial
3 = Extremely harmful	3 = Moderate	6 = Substantial	9 = Intolerable

Figure 5.4 3 × 3 risk matrix

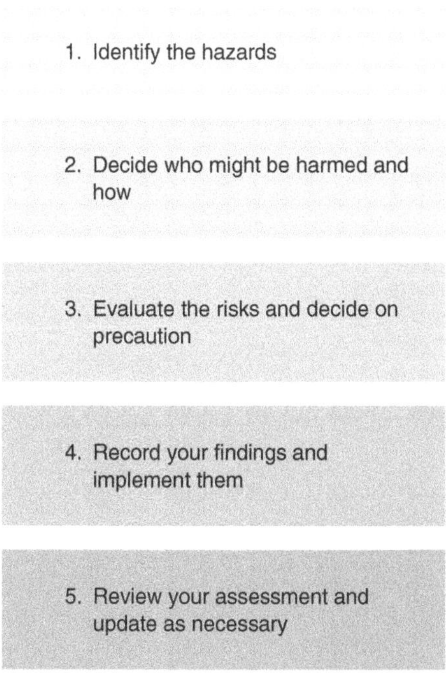

1. Identify the hazards

2. Decide who might be harmed and how

3. Evaluate the risks and decide on precaution

4. Record your findings and implement them

5. Review your assessment and update as necessary

Figure 5.5 Five steps in risk assessment

employee consultations and can alert managers to the potential hazard in their work area and the need to review the current risk assessment and risk controls.

The process of risk assessment can be followed using the five steps in risk assessment (Figure 5.5).

However the complexity of the risk assessment will vary enormously depending on what is being assessed. Some may be managed at local level, others may require the employment of specialists – engineers, chemists, risk managers or safety advisers.

Health surveillance acts as a check and audit of the risk management plan according to Hawley.[23] He states that flowing from the risk assessment will be a strategy for risk management which will seek to remove the hazard or, failing that, to control it. This can be achieved through engineering or procedural approaches. Figure 5.6 shows Hawley's flow chart for health surveillance.

Health surveillance and personal protective equipment

Where a hazard has been identified the onus is on the employer to prevent harm occurring or to ensure all reasonable effort has been made to reduce the risk of harm occurring. When considering control of hazard methods, there is a recognised hierarchy, and protecting the individual with personal equipment or clothing comes very much near the bottom. The Personal Protective Equipment Regulations 1999 (amended 2002)[24]

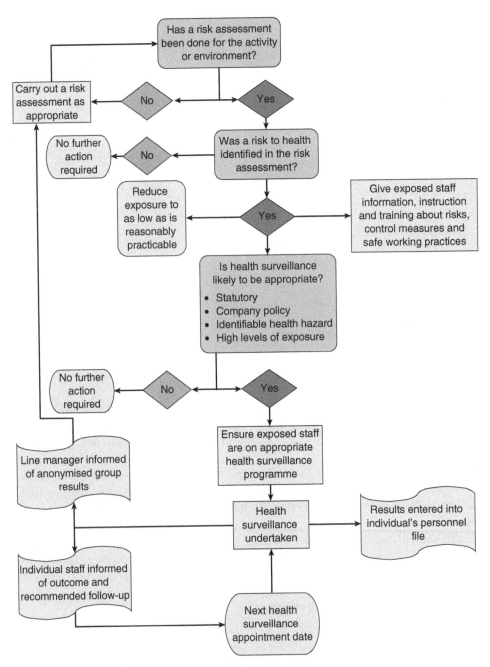

Figure 5.6 Flow chart for health surveillance

require that equipment is to be supplied and used at work wherever there is a risk to health and safety that cannot be adequately controlled in other ways. However, these regulations do not apply where there is other legislation with mandatory requirements for the provision and use of PPE in relation to specific hazards:

- lead
- ionising radiation
- asbestos
- hazardous substances
- noise.

Interestingly, those regulations are the same as the ones requiring health or medical surveillance! OH advisers therefore need to have knowledge of the types of PPE available for the specific hazards, as the provision and use (or misuse) can be critical in the assessment of the individual's health risk.

Provision of health surveillance

Many large organisations have an in-house OH service or access to one, so health surveillance programmes will be run by them. Smaller companies will usually rely on external providers to run their surveillance, which may be one provider for all surveillance required or multiple suppliers. Sole-trading OH advisers may offer as part of their contract with a company to be the responsible person to manage the provision and coordinate the different schemes, and manage the reporting and records. Either way, it is vital that there is effective communication between OH professionals and health and safety managers. Tim South[25] states that a lack of communication can lead to the OH department collecting information which charts the progress of damage to employees' health, while those responsible for the management of health and safety fail to intervene to prevent it. This is not good for either employees' health and welfare or for the long-term financial prospects of the employer.

Suitable health surveillance

Audiometry

Hearing damage caused by exposure to noise at work is permanent and incurable. It is usually gradual due to prolonged exposure to noise and with the effects of normal ageing loss can result in deafness. The law requires employers to assess the risks to their employees from noise at work, take action to reduce the noise exposure that produces those risks, provide their employees with hearing protection if the noise exposure cannot be reduced by other means, make sure the legal limits are not exceeded, provide employees with information, instruction and training and carry out health surveillance where there is a risk to health. Occupations where noise may be a hazard can be seen in Figure 5.7.

Hearing health surveillance requires equipment and procedures. The process of testing hearing ability is called audiometry, and the instrument to test is an audiometer. The procedure for hearing surveillance should be written up and will include reference to the noise risk assessment, the exposed groups of workers and the procedure for

Engineering	Farming	Paper and board manufacture
Demolition	Road building/repair	Textile manufacture
Woodworking	Forging, pressing or stamping	Construction and fabrication
Canning and bottling	Music and entertainment	Bars and clubs
Foundries	Plastics processing	Forestry and logging
Railways	Boiler making	Airways and airports
Military	Gamekeeping	Merchant shipping and fishing

Figure 5.7 Occupations where noise exposure may be a hazard

using the information. The Health Surveillance Guidance on the Control of Noise at Work[26] has full details of the procedure for hearing health surveillance, which is also available online.

The procedure will usually be as follows:

- awareness and instruction for at-risk employees and information for managers
- baseline hearing health surveillance before the individual is exposed to loud noise:
  - o hearing history and health questionnaire
  - o otoscopic examination
  - o audiometric test

- annual review for 2 years:
  - o update answers to hearing questionnaire
  - o otoscopic examination
  - o audiometric test

- 3-yearly examinations thereafter.

More frequent testing may be required if significant changes in hearing level are detected or exposure changes.

Hand–arm vibration syndrome

Hand–arm vibration syndrome (HAVS), formerly known as vibration white finger, is caused by prolonged exposure of the hand–arm system to mechanical vibration, which can cause vascular, neurological and musculoskeletal injury. With repeated and prolonged exposure to vibration, the individual may experience intermittent attacks of spasm in the fingers causing the blood flow to stop and the affected area to turn white. This may last for up to 30 minutes initially, but as the condition worsens the attacks are more frequent and eventually can lead to the ulceration of the skin and gangrene (very similar to Raynaud's disease). Neurologically there is a progressive numbness and tingling in the fingers and joints with loss of sensation and consequent inability to have normal hand function. Vibration increases the likelihood of the individual developing a musculoskeletal disorder. It is estimated that about 5 million workers in the UK are exposed to vibration at work.

Common activities that can lead to HAVS include:

- operating hand-held power tools
- holding materials that are being processed by vibrating machines
- using hand-guided equipment that is vibrating.

The Guidance on Regulations[27] state that it is essential that health professionals involved in health surveillance for HAVS can demonstrate that they have the necessary expertise. Specialist training is required to carry out adequate clinical assessments and avoid misdiagnosing symptoms of HAVS. When health surveillance is required, it should be carried out annually. Both initial (or baseline) assessment and routine health surveillance are needed for HAVS. Early assessment of newly exposed workers is recommended, as susceptible individuals can develop symptoms in 6 months or less. Exposed workers should receive information on why and how to detect and report symptoms of HAVS. The surveillance should follow this pattern:

- self-administered questionnaire following instruction from OH professional:
  - o OH assessment of response
  - o self-reporting of symptoms
- annual screening questionnaire:
  - o OH assessment of response
  - o self-reporting of symptoms
- OH consultation after 3 years if no symptoms
- symptoms disclosed:
  - o clinical assessment
  - o formal diagnosis
  - o optional standardised tests.

Full guidance on the 'five-tier' health surveillance for HAV can be found on the HSE website.[28]

Lung function

Many occupational environments and processes can expose the employee to inhalable substances that can cause respiratory illness like rhinitis, asthma, chronic obstructive pulmonary disease, fibrosis, allergic alveolitis or malignancy. The substances can be in the form of aerosols, mists, dusts, fumes and smokes as well as gases and vapours. They are responsible for acute or chronic effects, immediate symptoms, irritations or sensitisation after repeated exposures; they can also damage other organs of the body. Exposure limit values (EH40)[29] for these agents are available to guide appropriate controls in the workplace. Statutory medical examination is required for those working with asbestos and lead, and health surveillance under COSHH. Figure 5.8 shows common respiratory sensitisers.

Lung function health surveillance will be carried out by a suitably qualified and competent person within the OH department who has a knowledge and understanding of the effects of respiratory irritants and sensitisers, and the technical aspects of respiratory function tests. The usual procedure is as follows:

- Animals and insects (droppings, urine, hair, fur, feathers, mites) in farming, veterinary, equine and kennels
- Flour, grain, hay, pollen from handling, milling, baking, malting
- Glues and resins
- Isocyanates (toluene, naphthalene, etc.) in soft cushioning foams, building insulation, vehicle paint sprays
- Latex
- Soldering/welding fluxes (rosin and colophony) in electronic assembly
- Wood dusts – sawing and sanding; use of MDF

Figure 5.8 Common respiratory sensitisers

- awareness and instruction to at-risk employees and information to managers
- baseline health surveillance preferably before exposure to inhalable substances or those identified as requiring respiratory protection, but within 3 months of employment in at-risk areas:

  o respiratory questionnaire
  o respiratory function test/spirometry

- 3-month review:

  o update answers to questionnaire
  o respiratory function

- 6-month review for first 2 years
- annual review thereafter if no problems identified
- if health issues raised then more frequent monitoring and referral to OH physician if individual meets the appropriate criteria.

Advice, information and instruction on respiratory health should be given to the employee at OH consultations.

Full guidance on respiratory health surveillance for different conditions and industries can be found on the HSE website.[30]

Skin assessment

The skin is the largest organ of the body and has many functions, one of which is to act as a protective barrier to the rest of the body. If this barrier is breached, then the body is vulnerable to attack from chemicals, infections and other injury. The commonest reaction is contact dermatitis, where the skin reacts locally by producing an inflammation – eczema, characterised by redness, swelling, blistering, flaking and cracking. Conditions include contact urticaria, oil acne (mineral oils), chloracne (aromatic hydrocarbons), ulcers (chrome acids), depigmentation (alkyl phenols) and skin cancer (coal tar products, mineral oils, ultraviolet radiation). Other skin-affecting substances include latex, epoxy resins, solvents, cleaning and degreasing products, metal working fluids, plant saps and wood dusts, enzymes, prolonged wet work, cement, soaps and detergents. If detected early enough and the worker's exposure is reduced, then many of these conditions are curable.

Skin can be damaged after just one exposure or after repeated exposures. Some substances can be irritant, where the skin produces an inflammatory reaction, or act as a sensitiser where the result is an allergic reaction, and future exposure to even a tiny amount can provoke a reaction. Regulation for this group of workers is covered by COSHH 1999 (2002)[4] and CHIP 2009.[11]

Skin health surveillance will be carried out by a suitably qualified and competent person within the OH department who has a knowledge and understanding of the effects of dermal irritants and sensitisers. The usual procedure is as follows:

- awareness and instruction to at-risk employees and information to managers
- baseline assessment of the individual's skin condition, preferably before exposure to substances known to cause skin problems or those identified as requiring hand or skin protection, but within 6 weeks of employment in at-risk areas
- assessment of individual's skin condition and record on skin inspection record:

  o skin health and exposures questionnaire
  o inspection of hands, forearms and other areas which might be contaminated

- instruction to the individual and responsible person within the work area to conduct regular inspections and report to OH any symptoms between examinations.

The health surveillance may provide early warning of lapses in control and indicate the need for a reassessment of the risk.

Health surveillance and medical surveillance

The COSHH Regulations 1999 (2002) state that:

> **11** (5) If an employee is exposed to a substance specified in Schedule 6 and is engaged in a process specified therein, the health surveillance required under paragraph (1) shall include medical surveillance under the supervision of a relevant doctor at intervals of not more than 12 months or at such shorter intervals as the relevant doctor may require.

Figure 5.9 lists the substances in Schedule 6.
Other legislation where medical surveillance is stipulated:

- Asbestos at Work 2002[7] 22 (c): 'Each employee who is exposed to asbestos is under adequate medical surveillance by a relevant doctor.'
- Lead at Work 2002:[6] 10 (1): 'Every employer shall ensure that each of his employees who is or is liable to be exposed to lead is under suitable medical surveillance by a relevant doctor.'
- Ionising Radiation 1999:[10] 4 (2): 'The employer shall ensure that each of his employees to whom this regulation relates is under adequate medical surveillance

Vinyl chloride monomer (VCM)
Nitro or amino derivatives of phenol and of benzene or its homologues
Potassium or sodium chromate or dichromate
Ortho-tolidine and its salts Dianisidine and its salts Dichlorobenzidine and its salts
Auramine Magenta
Carbon disulphide Disulphur dichloride Benzene, including benzol Carbon tetrachloride Trichlorethylene
Pitch

Figure 5.9 The list of substances in Schedule 6 of Control of Substances Hazardous to Health Regulations 1999 (2002).

Source: The Control of Substances Hazardous to Health Regulations 1999 (2002). Available online at: http://www.legislation.gov.uk/uksi/2002/2677/contents/made.

by an appointed doctor or employment medical adviser for the purpose of determining the fitness of each employee for the work with ionising radiation which he is to carry out.'

The appointed doctor – in practice usually an occupational physician – will conduct a baseline and then regular clinical examination of at-risk individuals and any tests that may be required to ascertain their health, e.g. blood and urine tests for lead levels. The doctor must decide on the fitness of the individual to continue working in the exposed environment and certify any entry on the health record. Each regulation where medical surveillance is required gives detailed information on the full remit of the doctor, particularly regarding health records, asbestos licences and notification to the HSE. The doctor will also be involved in advising the employer on the future employment of an individual who is found to have an identifiable disease, in alternative work. COSHH 1999 (2002)[4] stipulates:

11 (6) Where an employee is subject to medical surveillance in accordance with paragraph (5) and a relevant doctor has certified by an entry in the health record of that employee that in his professional opinion that employee should not be engaged in work which exposes him to that substance or that he should only be so engaged under conditions specified in the record, the employer shall not permit the employee to be engaged in such work except in accordance with the conditions, if any, specified in the health record, unless that entry has been cancelled by a relevant doctor.

Who carries out health surveillance?

The COSHH Regulations 1999 (2002)[4] (**11** (12)) require certain roles in health and medical surveillance:

1. 'Appointed doctor' is a registered medical practitioner who is appointed for the time being in writing by the HSE for the purpose of this regulation. There is also a legal requirement for employees exposed to lead, asbestos and ionising radiation at work to have regular health checks carried out by an approved doctor.
2. 'Employment medical adviser' means an employment medical adviser appointed under section 56 of the Health and Safety at Work etc. Act 1974.[31]

Otherwise most health surveillance programmes are run and managed by OH advisers.

Health surveillance guidance[32] suggests that health surveillance in its simplest form involves employees checking themselves for signs or symptoms of ill health. The caveat is that it must be part of a health surveillance programme and in circumstances where the employee has been trained in what to look for and informed who to report symptoms to. The OH provider/adviser will need to demonstrate that he or she has the training and experience necessary to be able to set up a health surveillance programme, provide suitably qualified and experienced staff to carry out the work, be able to use and maintain any equipment necessary and provide the appropriate reports on employee fitness to enable the employer to conduct business.

The OH nurse adviser will:

- liaise with managers and safety in identifying the hazard and the risk and identify the employees exposed
- agree with the manager and staff representatives on what health surveillance is appropriate
- arrange for the exposed group to receive education and be able to self-question and self-examine depending on hazard, and know when to refer to OH
- arrange for statutory medical examination if required
- arrange for health-screening schedules and appointments
- conduct screening
- manage the administration of the programme
- write individual reports and group statistical reports, and maintain the health record
- follow up with individuals.

In some OH settings an OH support worker (OHSW) is employed. An OHSW has been defined by the Royal College of Nursing[33] as an individual who delivers OH services to and for individuals and groups. The OHSW will have the required level of knowledge and skills to recognise the influence of work on health, and will work under professional supervision within the guidance of established protocols and procedures. The OHSW will perform agreed health screening and surveillance, which can include education and collection of screening data arising from worker activity.

The OH physician will conduct the statutory medical examinations, and can advise on the results of health screening. The details of the legal requirements of the doctor in health and medical surveillance can be found in the specific regulations. According to new guidance from the British Medical Association,[2] part of the role is to monitor the health of workers who are potentially exposed to hazards at work through health surveillance programmes and analyse data from surveillance programmes using sound epidemiological methods to identify trends in worker health and recommend any remedial measures necessary to improve worker health. They can also be available for opinion on referral to specialists.

An occupational hygienist may also form part of the OH team. The International Occupational Hygiene Association defines occupational hygiene[34] as: 'The discipline of anticipating, recognizing, evaluating and controlling health hazards in the working environment with the objective of protecting worker health and well-being and safeguarding the community at large.' Occupational hygienists are specialists in the measurement of the personal exposure of a worker to the hazard/agent in the workplace, particularly at the relevant interface between the environment and the body, e.g. breathing zone, hearing zone and assessment of the data in terms of recommended workplace exposure limits, where such criteria exist.

OH teams will need to work very closely with safety professionals to have a coordinated approach to advising the employer in managing the occupational and safety risks in the organisation. The safety adviser will be able to offer assistance on assessing the hazard and risks and provide information on workplace inspections and alert OH if there is a problem that may need a health follow-up. The OH adviser can provide information on a potential workplace problem if a health issue is reported to him or her and alert management.

Records

The health record is not the same as the medical record. The health record is the non-confidential record of individuals' exposure to substances or physical hazards which may be harmful to their health and the health tests, procedures and examinations they have undertaken as part of health surveillance. It is a statutory requirement under the various regulations for an employer to hold such a record. The health record, as part of the health surveillance programme, will contain personal information, so it still needs to be stored securely and be accessed only by those who need to know; it is also subject to data protection legislation and should be kept by the employer. Under the Data Protection Act 1998,[13] employees have to be informed that a health record for them exists, and they have a right to access the information and correct it as necessary. Health records should be held by and be available to managers even when separate occupational medical records are also kept. However, sometimes they are held in OH departments, but need to be accessible by managers when required and it is therefore advisable to keep them separate from the individual's medical records. The health record needs to be kept for 40 years from the date of the last entry. All clinical information from medical consultations, test results, examinations and OH adviser assessments, reports and referral letters are to be kept in the individual's personal medical file.

The HSE advises that health records allow outcome analysis of ill health, in relation to exposure at a later stage, should this prove necessary (required under Regulation 5 of Management of Health and Safety at Work Regulations 1999,[3] the duty on employers to monitor and review their control measures). The HSE website has templates for the specific medical surveillances which can be adapted for an organisation. For general use the form must include the following:

- the name and address of the employer
- the name and address of the employee
- the employee's date of birth, gender, employee number, national insurance number
- date the employee started work in the organisation
- nature of employment
- details of work exposure in current employment
- details of any exposure in previous employment
- information on health surveillance carried out
- date and result of health surveillance fit, restrictions, unfit
- date, signature and status of practitioner.

The health record has to be kept for 40 years after the last entry. An example of a health record for general health surveillance is shown in Figure 5.10.

Health surveillance results

Where the health surveillance shows an employee has an identifiable disease or adverse health effect which is considered by a doctor (or in consultation with a doctor) to be the result of exposure to a hazardous substance or activity then the manager will be notified. The manager is then responsible for reviewing the risk assessment and any control measures and improving where practical. The OH practitioner will notify the employee and provide him or her with any relevant information and advice regarding future health surveillance and how to manage health. This may require referral to the general practitioner or hospital specialist. In discussion with the employee, the employer and staff representative, the individual may need to be assigned to different work to avoid or reduce exposure to the hazard.

Analysis of an exposed group's health surveillance results can be written up in the form of a statistical report for management which can be used to gauge the effectiveness of control measures. This information can also be made available to the employees and staff representatives.

Conclusion

Health surveillance is a core activity in OH and is used as a process of systematically watching for early signs of work-related ill health in employees exposed to certain

Surname:	First name:	Gender:	DOB:
Employee ID:	Nat Ins No:	Address:	
Occupation:			

Employer's name:

Place of work/Department:

Since:

Hazardous exposures (please give details):

- ☐ CBRN
- ☐ Noise
- ☐ Respiratory irritants/sensitisers
- ☐ Skin irritants/sensitisers
- ☐ Lead
- ☐ Chemical
- ☐ Biological
- ☐ Other

Work history:

Previous hazard exposures:

Date:	Health surveillance procedure:
Conclusion:	Fit/Fit with restrictions/Unfit. Comments
Examiner:	Signature & qualifications:
Date:	Health surveillance procedure
Conclusion:	Fit/Fit with restrictions/Unfit. Comments
Examiner:	Signature & qualifications
Date:	Health surveillance procedure:
Conclusion:	Fit/Fit with restrictions/Unfit. Comments
Examiner:	Signature & qualifications:
Date:	Health surveillance procedure
Conclusion:	Fit/Fit with restrictions/Unfit. Comments
Examiner:	Signature & qualifications
Date:	Health surveillance procedure:
Conclusion:	Fit/Fit with restrictions/ Unfit. Comments
Examiner:	Signature & qualifications:

Figure 5.10 An example of a health surveillance record

health risks. In many settings there is a statutory requirement to undertake health and/or medical surveillance and to keep appropriate records for 40 years after the last entry, but it can also be introduced if a particular health risk is identified. It is primarily aimed at prevention and starts with a risk assessment of the hazard, who might be harmed and how. It usually involves a set of questions and standardised tests and examinations of individuals in a selected exposed group. It is also an opportunity for the employer and employees to be informed and instructed in the hazard, risk controls and health consequences. Those who show signs of health issues can be readily identified and measures put in place to prevent further harm.

It is vital, with any health surveillance programme, to ensure that all participants are in full understanding of what it entails and what happens to the results. This will include the employer and the selected employees, the staff representatives and the individual managers, as well as the OH team, safety and hygienists. Trends in ill health or emerging patterns in workplace hazards can be demonstrated by health surveillance data. To be effective, surveillance has to be followed by preventive action and an evaluation of the effectiveness of intervention.[16]

References

1 International Labour Organization (1998) *Technical and Ethical Guidelines for Workers' Health Surveillance*. Geneva: ILO.
2 British Medical Association (2013) *The Occupational Physician*. London: BMA.
3 The Management of Health and Safety at Work Regulations 1999. Available online at: http://www.legislation.gov.uk/uksi/1999/3242/contents/made.
4 The Control of Substances Hazardous to Health Regulations 1999 (2002). Available online at: http://www.legislation.gov.uk/uksi/2002/2677/contents/made.
5 The Coal Mines (Control of Inhalable Dust) Regulations 2007. Available online at: http://www.legislation.gov.uk/uksi/2007/1894/contents/made.
6 The Control of Lead at Work Regulations 2002. Available online at: http://www.legislation.gov.uk/uksi/2002/2676/contents/made.
7 The Control of Asbestos at Work Regulations 2002. Available online at: http://www.legislation.gov.uk/uksi/2002/2675/contents/made.
8 The Control of Noise at Work Regulations 2005. Available online at: http://www.legislation.gov.uk/uksi/2005/1643/contents/made.
9 The Control of Vibration at Work Regulations 2005. Available online at: http://www.legislation.gov.uk/uksi/2005/1093/contents/made.
10 The Ionising Radiation at Work Regulations 1999 and associated Regulations. Available online at: http://www.legislation.gov.uk/uksi/1999/3232/contents/made.
11 The Chemicals (Hazard Information and Packaging for Supply) Regulations 2009. Available online at: http://www.legislation.gov.uk/uksi/2009/716/contents/made.
12 The Registration, Evaluation, Authorisation and Restriction of Chemicals 2007. Available online at: http://www.hse.gov.uk/reach.
13 Data Protection Act 1998. Available online at: http://www.legislation.gov.uk/ukpga/1998/29/contents.
14 Fischhoff B, Lichtenstein S, Slovic P, Derby SL, Keeny RL (1981) *Acceptable Risk*. Cambridge: Cambridge University Press.
15 Fewtrell L, Bartram J (eds) (2001) *Water Quality: Guidelines, standards and health*. London: World Health Organization.

16 Hoh D, Aw T-C (2003) Surveillance in OH. *Occup Environ Med* 60: 705–710.

17 Lewis J, Thornbory G (2012) *Employment Law and OH*. Chichester: Wiley Blackwell.

18 Kloss D (2010) *Occupational Health Law*. Oxford: Wiley.

19 Kloss D, Ballard J (2012) *Discrimination Law and OH Practice*. London: The At Work Partnership.

20 Black C, Frost D (2011) *Health at Work: An independent review of sickness absence*. London: HMSO.

21 Ministry of Justice *Pre-Action Protocol for Disease and Illness Claims*. Available online at: http://www.justice.gov.uk.

22 Reporting of Injuries, Diseases and Dangerous Occurrences Regulations 1995. Available online at: http://www.legislation.gov.uk/uksi/1995/3163/contents/made.

23 Hawley A (1998) Health surveillance: An operational imperative? *J R Army Medical Corps* 144: 66–71.

24 The Personal Protective Equipment Regulations 1999 (amended 2002). Available online at: http://www.legislation.gov.uk/uksi/2002/1144/contents/made.

25 South T (2004) *Managing Noise and Vibration at Work*. Oxford: Elsevier Butterworth-Heinemann.

26 HSE Guidance on the Control of Noise at Work. HSE L 108 2005. Available online at: http://www.hse.gov.uk/guidance/index.htm.

27 HSE Guidance Control of Vibration at Work. HSE L 140 2005. Available online at: http://www.hse.gov.uk/guidance/index.htm.

28 Health Surveillance website, hand–arm vibration. Available online at: http://www.hse.gov.uk/vibration/hav/advicetoemployers/havocchealth.pdf.

29 Workplace exposure limits (EH40). Available online at: http://www.hse.gov.uk/pubns/books/eh40.htm.

30 Lung function surveillance. Available online at: http://www.hse.gov.uk/lung-disease/index.htm.

31 HM Government (1974) The Health and Safety at Work etc. Act 1974. London: HMSO. Available online at: http://www.legislation.gov.uk/ukpga/1974/37.

32 HSE *Understanding Health Surveillance at Work*. HSE Indg304 and HSE website. Available online at: http://www.hsegov.uk/health-surveillance/index.htm.

33 Royal College of Nursing (2011) *Roles and Responsibilities of OH Support Workers*. London: RCN. Available online at: http://www.rcn.org.uk/__data/assets/pdf_file/0011/409439/004124.pdf.

34 International Occupational Hygiene Association. Available online at: http://www.ioha.net/faqs.html.

6

Health assessment, case management and rehabilitation

Susanna Everton, Sarah Mogford, Diane Romano-Woodward and Greta Thornbory

---

Learning objectives

After reading this chapter you will be able to:

- discuss the relevant employment legislation relating to absence management
- identify what knowledge and skills are necessary for undertaking a health assessment, functional assessment and case management in an occupational health (OH) setting
- appreciate the role of OH and take an active part in absence management policies and procedures
- appreciate the skills needed for professional report writing
- discuss critically the OH nurse's role in vocational rehabilitation.

Health assessment, case management and rehabilitation are all vital activities in OH nursing practice. The skills required to undertake this aspect of nursing are not included in all UK preregistration nurse training programmes and certainly not in the OH setting outside the national healthcare system. This chapter aims to explore comprehensively how health assessment in its various forms is undertaken for the benefit of both the employer and the employee. This is required under UK law, under the Health and Safety at Work Act etc. 1974, where it states that it is the duty of every employer to take reasonable care of the health, safety and welfare of all his employees and under the Equality Act 2010, which requires reasonable adjustments to be made by all employers for those with disabilities. More details of the legal aspects of OH practice can be found in the books by Lewis and Thornbory,[1] Kloss[2] and Kloss and Ballard.[3] These books are written by lawyers and explain the legal aspects of OH practice in depth.

> A health assessment may be defined as a one to one interaction between a client or employee and an occupational health professional, usually a doctor or a nurse, for the purposes of assessing the physical and/or mental health status of a client for employment purposes.[4]

Health assessments in OH need to be undertaken for a number of reasons:

- following an offer of, or change of employment, to check that the health of the applicant will not be adversely affected by the work and to assess whether any adjustments are necessary
- following a period of sickness absence when an employee is referred to OH, again to check that the employee would not be adversely affected by the work and to assess whether any adjustments are necessary
- when a referral is made by management to assess whether an employee has a medical condition which affects the employee's ability to give regular attendance at work or which may need adjustments
- under certain legislation following risk assessment. For example, where an individual may be exposed to a hazard, the health assessment for health surveillance establishes a baseline and a system to facilitate early detection of exposure/risk-related symptoms and allows action to prevent long-term health problems. More detailed information on health surveillance is given in Chapter 5
- for some jobs there are specific legislative requirements for either meeting medical standards or a prescribed structure of timed medical checks when a health assessment is necessary, e.g. pilots, divers, working with rail, offshore workers and driving (including heavy goods vehicles and passenger carriers).

Adjustments will be explored later in the chapter when dealing with rehabilitation, but meanwhile let us consider the actual health assessment. Again, taking a history and making a functional assessment is not something that is taught in preregistration training.[5]

The OH setting is different from many other clinical settings where nurses practise, in that the role is primarily to establish whether an individual is 'fit' to undertake a prescribed role without hazard or risk to him- or herself or others. Some assessments such as health surveillance and medicals for specific job roles (e.g. divers, pilots) carry prescribed methods, tests and criteria, thus following the medical model of assessment; most OH activities do not. OH assessment requires the ability to follow the biopsychosocial model of assessment. The OH nurse uses knowledge of job demands, abilities of the individual and clinical knowledge of any health condition to reach a professional conclusion in order to advise employer and employee appropriately.

Traditional training for physicians within the medical model involves taking a history and using tests to establish a diagnosis and treatment and, as mentioned before, nurse training often does not include 'history taking', as within the hospital setting it isn't required. Within OH assessment, the individual's status is expressed or interpreted in functional terms in the context of job requirements as opposed to health condition, diagnosis, disability or impairment.[6] Therefore skills required for this, although appearing basic, need to be emphasised as the ability to take a history, effectively assess an individual and obtain all the information required for an OH assessment as a key component of the OH nurse role.

Basics required for OH assessment

An OH assessment may take place face to face or increasingly via telephone. In either circumstance, it is an interview-style situation for which the OH nurse needs to be prepared.

- Consent needs to be obtained. The individual should be informed and understand the purpose of the OH appointment, confidentiality, report process and consent status. Ideally the employee has been informed by the employer beforehand and best practice requires OH providers to publish clear information for service users. However, a key skill of the OH nurse is to establish rapport quickly to facilitate an effective assessment whilst informing and reassuring individuals who may not understand the purpose of the appointment; indeed, they may be fearful if this is part of a disciplinary procedure. Professional and legal obligations regarding both confidentiality and consent within OH can be complex and are discussed in Chapter 1. OH nurses should ensure they are fully conversant with both professional guidance and legal status. The 2009 General Medical Council Guidance on Confidentiality Paragraph 34 is a good summary.[7]
- OH nurses should be clear as to the purpose of the assessment. A management referral should indicate the areas that require OH advice and ask specific questions that require answers. Employees should also be aware of the questions being asked, not just from a consent issue, but also as this is a dialogue and assessment of them. There is more cooperation if employees feel that they are involved with the process.
- Clinical records, whether manual notes or computerised records, should comply with the relevant legislation and professional guidelines and more details are given on this aspect at the end of the chapter.
- Environment – if the assessment is being carried out by telephone, the employee's identity must be established and confidentiality maintained (i.e. the employee should be in a place where he or she cannot be overheard and can speak freely). Any interview room needs to be appropriate for the role and ensure privacy. This includes any equipment, assessment tools or forms required.
- Observational, interviewing and clinical assessment skills need to be honed as part of the process. On arrival the OH nurse should take note of factors such as: is the employee out of breath? Is the individual able to move with ease, take a coat off, get in/out of a chair?
- Resulting report – this is covered further later in this chapter.

Functional assessment

The terms functional assessment and vocational rehabilitation are often used. Functional assessment is assessing the basic functional components of the individual, task and/or role. Vocational rehabilitation is using activity (often the workplace) as rehabilitation. Rehabilitation will be addressed later in this chapter.

The usual nursing assessment framework of activities of daily living[8] is of limited use in workplace function, but using domestic/social activities as a comparison for job function and stamina is useful when considering the physical functional assessment. These can be described as 'instrumental activities of daily living'[9] and can include phone use, managing finances, shopping, housework and driving. Basic psychological assessments can also use comparators – how the individual is managing the stresses of everyday life and using tools such as the Hospital Anxiety and Depression Scale.[10]

Key to the functional assessment is the OH nurse having an effective understanding of the individual's functions and job role and being able to break these down, equate and assess an individual's particular circumstances. Considering the impact of sustaining a task (including stamina issues) is important. One of the main criticisms of the Department for Work and Pensions Capability Assessment is that sustainability of individual action/function isn't considered.[11] There are many models for more formal physical and psychological functional assessments with tasks replicating work functions and individuals are measured for one function (e.g. sitting) – how long, how often – before they can repeat such a task. Specialist independent companies, often occupational therapist-led, offer both physical and psychological functional testing to a far higher intensity than would be expected within the average OH appointment time; they use detailed functional assessment tools such as the Saunders method[12] and Matheson system.[13]

The OH nurse can undertake an assessment of the individual's abilities to undertake a specific work role and advise on any limitations and role adjustments. However, OH nurses need to be aware of their own limitations and be able to identify when to obtain further information or when to refer on.

Absence management

Assisting management of an organisation in managing absence is key to the success of any OH service.

According to Miles Templeman, Director General of the Institute of Directors:[14]

> All enterprises seek to be in a healthy state. If employees are in a good state of health and wellbeing then that must surely contribute to successful performance? The downside of that is when time and effort is lost through sickness and other absence from work, or when employees are not getting or giving of their best.

It should not be forgotten that managing absence is a management responsibility and so management ought to be aware of the cost to the business of unplanned absences. There are various reasons why employees may be absent from work and statistics on this are gathered by a number of organisations. There are two significant annual business absence surveys undertaken, one by the Confederation of British Industry (CBI)[15] and the other by the Chartered Institute of Personnel and Development[16] (CIPD). Other work-related absence statistics are collated and published by the Health and Safety Executive (HSE).[17] It is worth taking some time to read the latest of these surveys as they are published annually. Viewing the different years gives one the trends in reasons for absence as well as the fluctuation in numbers. At times of economic difficulties when people are being laid off then sickness absence reduces whilst at good economic times sickness absence rises. Both the CIPD and CBI surveys give the figures and costs and the interventions that have proved most beneficial for reducing absence and year on year they have stated that, along with return-to-work interviews (RTWIs), OH involvement is the most effective method of dealing with long-term absence.

Employees are expected to attend work in order to carry out their duties and it is reasonable for employers to expect regular attendance and good time keeping. In the UK employers are required by law to provide an employee with a 'written statement of employment' and the principal statement can be seen in Box 6.1.

Box 6.1   Written statement of employment requirements under Employment Rights Act 1966

Most employees are legally entitled to a written statement of the main terms and conditions of employment within two calendar months of starting work – this should include:

- Employee's and employer's name
- Employee job title or a brief job description
- Date when the employment began
- Pay rate and when it will be paid
- Hours of work
- Holiday entitlement
- Where the employee will be working (if based in more than one place, it should say this, along with the employer's address)
- Sick pay arrangements
- Notice periods
- Information about disciplinary and grievance procedures
- Any collective agreements that affect employment terms or conditions
- Pensions and pension schemes
- If not a permanent employee, how long the employment is expected to continue, or if a fixed-term worker the date employment will end

---

Source: www.acas.org.uk.

Therefore employees are expected to fulfil their part of the written statement. However there are a number of planned reasons, as well as unplanned reasons, why an employee may not be at work, as can be seen from Table 6.1. Managers are able to arrange planned absences at a local level and take account of them as part of departmental management and this includes planned sickness absence such as elective surgery. However, managers encounter problems when employees take unplanned leave. This

Table 6.1 Planned and unplanned absences from work

Planned	Unplanned
Annual leave	Military service
Study leave	Jury service
Maternity/paternity	Bereavement/compassionate leave
Time off in lieu	Unplanned health problems
Sabbatical/break in service	
Planned healthcare	
Trade union duties	

is singly the biggest cost to employers, especially in terms of minor illness – generally this is regarded as less than 4 weeks and it is mainly in the realm of fewer than 7 days.

The CBI report[15] states that one-third of employers believe that non-genuine sickness absences occur across their organisation. Often there are reasons why sick leave is taken, such as family reasons, a sick child or relative, and this is a factor that needs to be addressed with family-friendly policies and carers' leave.

For some years now these annual surveys and reports have shown that the main reasons for long-term absence, i.e. over 4 weeks, are musculoskeletal disorders and mental ill health related to stress, anxiety and depression. It is especially in these areas that rehabilitation needs to be considered as one of the main strategies for dealing with absence management. Chapter 7 on mental health deals with this area in depth.

Measuring and recording absence

Management need to keep accurate records of absences from work and to be able to calculate statistics for monitoring absence levels and the reasons for absences.[18] The CIPD factsheet on Absence Measurement and Management[18] gives clear guidelines on the different ways of measuring absence, including the Bradford score, which is the most well-known tool, although not necessarily the most popular or efficient (Box 6.2). It is a good idea for all OH nurses to understand what systems are used, but to remember that it is management's job, and not the OH department's, to keep this information.

Some organisations now use computerised systems which will include a complete sickness absence/management referral/OH system. These software systems can monitor the sickness/absence of staff and clients and will recognise repetitive periods of sickness, highlighting trends and bringing to attention problem cases. The programmes include a comprehensive reporting tool, empowering the company to produce any sickness absence reports as required:

- proactive approach to sickness absence
- Bradford score enabled
- spells of absence recorded
- certification type catered for.

Box 6.2   The Bradford factor score

The Bradford factor score is an index of absence for individuals in an organisation, which gives more weight to the number of spells of absence within a given period than to their duration and determines when these have become excessive. It was first proposed by Bradford University during a series of lectures on production management in the 1980s. It is difficult to identify the research or evidence upon which it is based.

The formula is usually applied over a period covering the last 52 weeks, although other periods could be used. Frequent short absences will produce a higher Bradford factor score than less frequent absences with the same number of days off. This can be used by organisations as a trigger point for action. Note that it should be used only as part of a comprehensive attendance management policy and procedures, and not in isolation. The circumstances leading to a high score should be discussed with the individual prior to any action being taken. If the individual has a condition which might be considered a disability under the Equality Act 2010, then the accommodation which might be considered by management would be to allow a higher Bradford factor score before action is taken. Alternatively, absence associated with disability or pregnancy-related absence can be excluded from the calculation.

The calculation for the Bradford factor (B) is number of occasions sick (S) × number of occasions sick (S) × total number of days absent (D) or

$$B = S^2 \times D$$

Typical thresholds are:

0–49	No action required
50–124	Consider issuing a verbal warning
125–399	Consider issuing a first written warning
400–649	Consider issuing a final written warning
650+	Consider dismissal

For example, if an employee is off sick five times each for one day at a time then:

$$B = 5 \times 5 \times 5 = 125$$ and it would be time to issue a first written warning.

Sources: http://employmentlawclinic.com/attendance-and-performance/bradford-factor; http://www.orbuk.org.uk/article/the-bradford-factor.

Table 6.2 Factors affecting sickness absence

Macro level	Organisational level	Individual level
• Climate	• Nature of the industry	• Age
• Epidemics	• Working conditions	• Gender
• Provision of healthcare services	• Job demands	• Occupational status
• Social insurance systems	• Size of the enterprise	• Job satisfaction
• Sickness certification practices	• Characteristics of the workforce	• Length of service
• Taxation	• Workforce availability	• Personality
• Pensionable age	• Industrial relations	• Life crises
• Social attitudes	• Supervisory quality	• Family responsibility
• Economic climate	• Personnel policies	• Social support
• Available alternative employment	• Labour turnover	• Leisure activities
• Unemployment	• The provision of occupational health services	• Alcohol intake
		• The health status of the individual

Source: Whitaker SC (2001) The management of sickness absence. *Occup Environ Med* 58 (6): 420–424. Available online at: http://oem.bmj.com/content/58/6/420.full (accessed 26.04.13).

It has been shown in the CIPD[16] and CBI[15] reports that the earlier OH are involved with employees on long-term sick leave, then the easier it is to implement a return to work. Most organisations have trigger points for referral within their sickness absence policies and procedures and these are usually when sickness absence has reached 15 or 21 days.

Factors that affect sickness absence

The factors that affect sickness absence can be seen in Table 6.2.[19]

Absence management: policies and procedures

Employees need to know what is expected of them and their line managers need to know and understand absence management and the difference between planned and unplanned absence. The CBI states that good absence management needs commitment from the top and having the right policies in place is paramount.[15] The policy and procedures for absence management, including sickness absence, should be clearly laid out for everyone in the organisation and easily understood as well as widely accepted.

Developing absence management policies and procedures

All stakeholders need to be involved in the development of policies and procedures and that includes:

- human resources (HR)
- managers, particularly line managers
- employees, possibly through their representatives and/or the trade unions
- OH professionals who can give advice and guidance and may have to conduct statutory health assessments and medical examinations.

When preparing the policy, it should include all the aspects of managing an employee's absence from work, both planned and unplanned, and all the necessary aspects of return to work.

Some organisations prefer today to look at the title of absence management policies with a more positive note and call them 'attendance' policies and procedures rather than the negative-sounding 'absence'. Other factors to consider are the gathering of absence statistics and the procedures for keeping and analysing them so that they produce meaningful figures for the company. There need to be clear procedures for both managers and employees so they will be aware of the roles and functions of those dealing with absence, with definite statements so people know the trigger points for putting management action into play, such as the number of days off or absences allowed in a given period or the cause of the absence, e.g. workplace accident, before management action would be instigated.

The HSE website[20] gives plenty of guidance on dealing with sickness absence, as does the Advisory Conciliation and Arbitration Service (ACAS)[21] and CIPD; they also offer sample policy and procedures for managing absence. CIPD[22] offers a sample policy and guidance and state that an effective absence policy should encompass the following key elements:

- a clear statement of the standards of attendance expected by the organisation
- explicit management commitment to the organisation's absence policies, standards and procedures
- systematic procedures for managing absence
- systematic procedures for investigating and managing 'problem' absence.

Reporting absence

If managers are to manage then they need to know when someone is unable to attend for work. This makes reporting absence one of the key procedures for managing the workforce. Each company will need an appropriate reporting procedure; it should state who employees should inform of their absence and when, and the frequency of reporting where necessary. Some jobs are time-critical and an employee not following correct procedures can cause problems for the business, resulting in loss of business or diminished quality of service. If the company procedures say that the employer needs to be notified 1 hour before a shift commences and the employee does not phone in until half-way through the shift then the employer is not able to make suitable arrangements for cover. In these days of easy communication by mobile phone and email there is less excuse than in the past when people maybe had to leave the house to find a phone – not easy if one is feeling ill. However, employers should always understand when an emergency occurs and people are unable to follow normal procedures.

The reporting policy needs to be clear what employees should do. It should be easily accessible to all and employees should be aware of the policy, together with warning that failure to follow these procedures could result in disciplinary proceedings; people will then be left in no doubt as to what is expected of them. Once the policy and procedures are in place then management can start to keep accurate statistics and monitor the levels of unplanned/unauthorised absence.

Included in the cost of unplanned absence the following should be taken into account: the cost of temporary staff, loss of customer goodwill, contracts and deadlines, poor service, low staff morale and stress placed on other members of the team.

The fit note

In the UK when employees go off sick for longer than 1 week they are expected to give the employer a note from the treating doctor. In the past this has been called the sick note or sick certificate, but the Black report[23] in 2008 recommended that this be reviewed and a new 'fit note' be introduced. The report made a number of recommendations concerning the health and wellbeing of Britain's working-age population and led to a major reform in the way in which UK general practitioners certified sickness absence.

The traditional medical statement or 'sick note' was replaced by the fit note in April 2010. The old sick note stated whether or not a patient was fit for work, whereas the fit note offers the doctor an option to say the person is fit for work with a phased return, amended duties, altered hours or workplace adaptations. The purpose of the fit note is to emphasise what employees can do rather than what they cannot do and full details for OH professionals are given in a government document.[24] A dilemma can occur for management when trying to accommodate the reduced attendance of an employee if the advice from the fit note is followed. The cost of covering a role for part hours/days may not be in the interest of the organisation and it may be that, despite the best of intentions, it is not possible to get an employee back to work sooner on a phased return. The OH adviser may be involved in these discussions and needs to be aware of the interests of the organisation as well as the 'patient'.

Return-to-work interviews

RTWIs, trigger mechanisms and the use of disciplinary procedures have been rated as the most effective approaches to deal with short-term absence according to both the CIPD[16] and CBI[15] surveys. In fact, the RTWI appears to be more effective than disciplinary measures and recommendations are that it should be carried out after every period of unscheduled absence. What is important is that the interviews are conducted sensitively as employees resent them if badly handled,[25] and that line managers receive the appropriate training to deal with absence management and in particular how to conduct the interview. There are apocryphal stories of managers reading from a prepared script and making apologies for this 'new management process they have to do'. ACAS is aware that managers are often not trained to take on a people management role and so offer online free training, including managing absence and guidance on the RTWI. This guidance is given here, not because it is the role of the OH nurse but first for information and second for those OH nurses who have a management role in the OH team.

An RTWI should consist of the following:

- Welcome back:
  - o Let the person know that he/she has been missed and that it is good to see him/her return, without making him/her feel guilty. Update him/her with any company or department news.
- Make enquiries:
  - o Find out the reason for the absence and ask if the individual feels well enough to work. Remember it is not right to explore the details of medical conditions; the employee may find this an invasion of privacy and medical details are sensitive information under the Data Protection Act. If the manager is concerned about the reason for sickness absence then the person should be referred to the OH service. It is at this stage that other factors may come to light, such as whether the absence is work-related; consideration must also be given to whether the employee has a disability under the Equality Act, which would require adjustments to be made. This might mean that a new risk assessment of the job or work environment is necessary and would require involvement of OH or health and safety team.
- Remind employee:
  - o If necessary at this stage the employee should be reminded of the expected level of attendance and notified as to how much time he/she has taken off as sickness absence.
- Offer assistance:
  - o The manager should always offer to assist the employee.
- Record:
  - o It is essential for management to keep a written record of the interview, complete with date, time and length.

Long-term absence

Evidence from all the surveys undertaken[15,9,16] demonstrates that providing the employer or manager has kept in touch with the employee then he/she will find it less difficult to return to work. It should be remembered that returning to work is a big step, especially after a major illness or operation, and may cause anxiety and bring on all sorts of health implications. Therefore it may be better to consider a phased return and assess whether any adjustments are needed. Rehabilitation will be dealt with later in this chapter, but should be based on sound professional advice from an OH nurse or doctor.

OH referral

Referral to OH must be a formal procedure. In the past managers have used OH as a threat and a disciplinary measure; subsequently employees then view OH as a management tool and are concerned about the confidentiality of their personal and medical details. However, that practice is dying out now that the public are more enlightened. OH professionals are still frustrated by the person who turns up to the department saying he/she has been sent by his/her manager without any idea why and no formal letter of referral. The OH nurse has no idea what management wants to know, so how can any decision be made without knowing the ins and outs of the employee's job and position? Besides which, even after having been seen and assessed by OH, there is no actual request for OH to send a report and the employee has not given his/her written consent to such. This is why the referral process should be included in the policy and procedures and it is better to use a proforma referral. A sample is given in Lewis and Thornbory.[1]

It should be remembered that the employee has signed consent and that he/she understands and agrees to an OH report being prepared in accordance with the employee's rights under the Data Protection Act. The 2009 guidance by the General Medical Council on confidentiality[26] also provides important information, as does the Faculty of Occupational Medicine.[27]

Once the formal request is received by the OH service then arrangements and an appointment can be made with the employee to be seen by the OH nurse or doctor. It is essential that the correct approach is taken and policies and procedures are followed. This is the key aspect that employment tribunals look for. The appeals tribunal judge, Mr J Wood, in the case of *Lynock* v *Cereal Packaging Ltd*,[28] stated: 'It is important to realise that these cases are not cases of disciplinary situations; what is important is that the employers should treat each case individually where there is genuine illness and with sympathy, understanding and compassion.' Lewis and Thornbory[1] say that this case remains a cornerstone for management's handling and best practice of sickness absence.

One of the aspects of health assessment for the OH nurse is triaging, in other words deciding whether the client needs to be seen by the OH nurse or doctor. This should be discussed with the doctor and a departmental policy devised. Certain management referrals, such as those where ill health retirement has to be considered, or where an employee has shown a lack of progress with a work-related condition, will usually need to be seen by the doctor. Most pension companies demand a medical report for ill-health retirement. These aspects of OH practice should be included in the Service Level Agreement (SLA) with the company and the key performance indicators (KPI) for the OH department. SLAs and KPIs will be discussed in depth in Chapter 8.

Case management

Case management has in the past been regarded as the domain of the community health professionals and there is a Case Management Society UK,[29] which states that the role of a case manager is to collaborate with clients by assessing, facilitating, planning and advocating health and social needs on an individual basis. The Department of Health is supporting the case management concept by helping local health communities achieve the targets for improving care for people with long-term conditions. However, OH doctors and nurses have always been seen as people who 'advise' rather than 'manage' cases, but case management is now viewed as one significant way to deal with absence and rehabilitation in the workplace.

The Case Management Society UK[29] defines case management as:

> A collaborative process which assesses plans, implements, co-ordinates, monitors and evaluates the options and services required to meet an individual's healthcare, educational and employment needs, using communication and available resources to promote quality cost effective outcomes.

It is worth taking some time to read the case management standards on the UK website.[29] Case managers need to be trained and skilled people but they are not necessarily healthcare professionals. Indeed, if you read the article about the Leicester fit for work pilots[30] you will see that the case managers are people from various professional backgrounds who are experienced in dealing with clients with employment and/or social problems. You will see from this work that management of clients' needs which affect their health and wellbeing extends beyond the disease, illness or medical condition itself. The social and psychological factors are extremely influential and need to be considered when dealing with absence management and rehabilitation. This is known as the biopsychosocial model of health.[31] Waddell and Burton comment that traditionally in the past doctors and nurses have always viewed the management of sickness absence and rehabilitation from the biomedical viewpoint but now the biopsychosocial model gives a far more rounded view of what affects the health and wellbeing of the client. It stands to reason then that the person who manages the client's case is able to explore the biopsychosocial aspects of the individual and this may or may not be a doctor or a nurse. So we need to consider the team aspect of case management: who are the stakeholders and who are the case management team?

These are examples of how working in a multidisciplinary team can help to deal with complex cases. Where needed, other services could have contributed to the case management team – such as Access to Work, employee assistance programme people, counsellors, cognitive behavioural therapists, occupational therapists or even one of the relevant charities. Decisions are not made in isolation but as part of a team effort, viewing all the aspects of the case. Case management can be a valuable tool for OH professionals in supporting employers and employees alike in the health and wellbeing of the workforce.

Vocational rehabilitation

At the launch of the Vocational Taskforce in July 2007, Lord McKenzie said:

> Rehabilitation is not about forcing people back to work. Work, in fact, is often a crucial step in helping people return to health. And businesses have much to gain in terms of reduced sickness absence, and improved staff engagement and retention.[32]

This statement has been backed up by the research undertaken by Waddell and Burton,[31,33] which has added to the body of knowledge on this topic. Both texts quote several pieces of research which say that many people can and do work with common health problems (and some not so common ones too!). They go on to say that better clinical and occupational management should minimise the impact on work performance and productivity. Work, in fact, is often a crucial step in helping people return to full health.

According to the Vocational Rehabilitation Association (VRA), vocational rehabilitation is a process which enables people with functional, psychological, developmental, cognitive and emotional impairments or health conditions to overcome barriers to accessing, maintaining or returning to employment or other useful occupation.[34]

Waddell and Burton demonstrated that work can be an effective part of the secondary or treatment stage of healthcare.[33] They go on to say that worklessness is strongly associated with poor mental and physical health, higher mortality, higher medical and hospital needs and low self-esteem. Conversely employment provides the opposite and it is said that better clinical and OH management and rehabilitation of common health problems are the best ways to deal with long-term sickness absence for the benefit of the employee as well as the employer, but it requires a multi- or interdisciplinary approach.

The VRA has standards which say that the rehabilitation process is interdisciplinary by nature, and may require functional, biopsychosocial, behavioural and/or vocational interventions; this fits in with the biopsychosocial model and the use of case management as a vital part of vocational rehabilitation. The VRA standards go on to list the techniques required for rehabilitation, although these are not exhaustive:

- assessment and appraisal
- goal setting and intervention planning
- provision of health advice and promotion, in support of returning to work
- support for self-management of health conditions
- career (vocational) counselling
- individual and group counselling focused on facilitating adjustments to the medical and psychosocial impact of disability
- case management, referral and service coordination
- programme evaluation and research
- interventions to remove environmental, employment and attitudinal obstacles
- consultation services among multiple parties and regulatory systems
- job analysis, job development and placement services, including assistance with employment

- job accommodations
- the provision of consultation about and access to rehabilitation technology.

These require appropriately trained and skilled people to deal with them and the VRA standards go on to lay down standards for practice in this area. OH nurses should be able to fulfil these criteria with the help and support of other relevant professionals as part of a multidisciplinary case management team.

A report on some pilot studies on rehabilitation research was published in 2006.[35] One of the key findings was that employees who had regular contact with line managers who had focused on the employees' health and wellbeing, rather than when they would be able to return to work, were generally more positive about returning to work. This is also borne out by the annual surveys by the CBI[15] and CIPD.[16]

The role of OH nurses in the rehabilitation of employees requires them to assess:

- the client by identifying the health problem and obtaining further medical information if necessary
- the workplace and possibly undertake or obtain a job analysis or risk assessment
- client's mode and time of travel to and from work
- client's access and egress in emergencies
- need for any ongoing treatment such as psychological or physical therapies where necessary
- the advice given to management, by means of a written report, any adjustments or restrictive duties where necessary.

Where restrictive duties on return to work are suggested, *Tolley's Guide to Employee Rehabilitation*[36] recommends a graduated or structured return to work such as a reduction of hours per day, working from home or carrying out partial duties. The authors also suggest that these are gradually increased over a period of 6–8 weeks maximum. They state that there is little point in returning to work for less than 4 hours per day, but in the first instance it may be worth the long-term absent employee returning for coffee, tea or lunch with colleagues to break the ice. Therapeutic interventions should take place outside these shorter working hours and the OH service should review the progress on a regular basis. It should not be a long-drawn-out process.

As musculoskeletal disorders are the commonest reasons for sickness absence it is worth reading the guidance by Kendall and Burton[37] on rehabilitating back to work people with these problems. It is based on the biopsychosocial model and uses the flag system.

Ill-health retirement

Where there is no prospect of a return to work the employer may have to look at terminating the employment with an early retirement on the grounds of ill health. If an employee could be entitled to an ill-health retirement pension then the employer must consider ill-health retirement before dismissing on incapacity grounds. The type of entitlement to ill-health retirement pension will depend on the organisation and in the case of the UK public sector this will differ from one body to another, so it is necessary for the OH service to be *au fait* with the type of ill-health retirement policy and the relevant criteria. An ill-health retirement is a situation where the employment is terminated, usually by voluntary resignation and mutual agreement. Pension insurance companies require there to be an assessment and report of the individual's medical condition recommending ill-health retirement, generally from a medical practitioner, as was mentioned previously. That report will then be considered by the company pension and/or any insurance scheme administrators for their decision.

Records and report writing

Writing a report is an integral part of OH nursing practice, but it is an area which is not always well performed or delivered. Many OH nurses do not appreciate that the report may be used as evidence in any legal situation within the workplace, and therefore, as a legal document, it needs to be well prepared, well presented and accurate. The report should also be written in such a way as to be easily understood by the recipient – usually the HR manager or line manager. The content of any OH report will contain as much information about the individual as is necessary to allow for the person to be managed successfully in the work environment, but that is also within the limits of the individual patient's confidentiality (see the section on confidentiality in Chapter 1). The OH nurse should respond to questions raised by management or HR to enable them to make appropriate adjustments for the employee or have an understanding of the likely course of his/her condition, but it is not required to divulge intimate health or medical details without the employee's consent or where not necessary. Nursing and Midwifery Council guidance on Codes of Practice[38] explains the OH role on consent. The Faculty of Occupational Medicine has stipulated in its *Good Occupational Medical Practice*[39] 'that the physician must be satisfied that, prior to a consultation or release of any information to employers or third parties, the worker consents to these proposed actions' and goes on to explain in detail how this applies. It is, therefore, considered good practice for OH nurses to follow this rule.

Types of occupational health reports

OH nurses will be required to write reports on different subjects relating to their practice:[1]

- employment fitness to work of an individual
- response to a management referral on an individual's fitness or work capability, including requirement, if any, for adjustments under Equality Act 2010[40]
- health surveillance reports
- workplace visit assessment
- business reports – financial cases, personnel, work activity etc.

When an OH nurse gives advice to an employer he or she will not normally refer to clinical details. The OH nurse may state that an employee is fit or unfit or that restrictions are required, and whether this is likely to be temporary or permanent. The employer does not need to know the clinical details behind that advice except with the written consent of the individual.

Management referrals

The management referral is central to the collaboration between the employer, employee and the OH service. It is advisable to have a standard format for a referral so that all the necessary information required to enable a suitable response from OH following consultation can be achieved. Any advice or guidance offered by OH should be based on the evidence and be unambiguous. It should be clear in the report where the information has come from:

- results of examinations/assessment
- results of tests
- reports from third parties, e.g. physiotherapists, cognitive therapists, specialists
- comments from line manager/HR
- opinion or testimony from the individual, e.g. 'the patient's account was as follows'.

Any report is information from an OH nurse to enable the line manager to make a decision about the individual. It is not the role of the OH nurse to make that decision for the manager. Figure 6.1 gives a template for a standard managerial report.

Medical in Confidence

Date:

To: Line manager
      HR manager

Re: [Insert employee's name, staff no. (if available), job title and department]

Thank you for referring [insert name] to occupational health for our opinion on:

[Write a brief paragraph on background and generalised content of consultation]

[Insert questions requested on the referral form and responses to them]

I am now able to inform you that:

- He/she is fit to carry out the full range of normal duties relating to his/her job
- He/she will be able to offer regular and efficient service
- He/she will probably be able to return to normal duties on [give date]
- He/she will probably be able to return to work subject to the following adjustments:

  [Insert adjustment advice]

- He/she is unfit to return to this post and would benefit from redeployment
- He/she is unfit to return to this post and we would support an application for retirement on ill health grounds
- Other [insert as appropriate]

Follow up appointment in [XX] weeks

Signed: _____

Date: _____

Name and designation: _____

Figure 6.1 Template for occupational health nurse report to management

Structure of report

The structure of the case report can be as follows and should be able to stand alone as an independent document and be read by another manager who may not be aware of the original referral (people move job roles!). Box 6.3 gives the items that would make up a structured report.[41]

Box 6.3   The structure of a management report

Write employee's full name, date of birth, employee number, job title and work area as reference.

Set the background in the introduction – who the employee is, what he/she does, for how long he/she has been doing it and a summary of the referral.

Summarise the consultation using non-confidential clinical information to outline the health issue and findings. (More details can be given if the individual has consented in the referral).

Explain how this health problem may interfere with the work activity – physical, psychological and environmental.

Answer the specific questions asked in the referral.

Consider your professional opinion on the fitness of the individual and if not fit or requiring work adjustments, explain how the situation can be improved; what treatment or further referral to specialists might be required; what adjustments in work activity or attendance might be required. Include an estimate on the time to give management a better opportunity to plan. Make a judgement on whether the work activity will delay or stop the individual's recovery. This is the unique position that occupational health professionals have over other health practitioners – they should know the work area!

Temporary adjustments can be suggested with a view to return to full work. If this is not a likely outcome, then the individual may require a reasonable adjustment under the Equality Act. It is important to remember that the occupational health adviser (OHA) is giving recommendations to the manager: it is up to the manager to decide if these can be accommodated in that area of work.

Ensure your statements are backed by evidence, e.g. the patient said . . . , on examination I found the following . . . , in my opinion . . . , the manager's opinion was . . . , the patient felt that . . . Often OHAs will find they are being used as a pawn between an employee and his or her manager and can find themselves under pressure to take sides.

The finishing comments should include that the contents have been discussed with the individual; if the individual has been referred externally, that a review is or is not required and when; or if the case is discharged. The manager is recommended to meet to discuss the outcomes with the employee.

Health surveillance report

Health surveillance is defined under the Control of Substances Hazardous to Health Regulations, Management of Health and Safety at Work Regulations and Control of Noise at Work Regulations (see Chapter 5).

- It should not be confused with general health screening or health promotion, as commonly used to look at lifestyle health issues.
- It follows from an identification of a health risk from an activity or exposure risk assessment.
- The health record is a record for an individual and is held by the manager. It should not include any clinical information, but should include the OH practitioner's conclusions on the employee's fitness for work.
- The General Health Surveillance Report to management is a statistical report based on the group of 'at-risk' employees. The results of tests and questionnaires are anonymously collated and analysed to produce a general view of employee health in relation to the work activity and exposure to harmful substances or hazards. This gives the manager an indication of the efficacy of the control measures in place (Figure 6.2).
- Where an individual shows changes which need to be alerted to the manager to protect the individual from further damage to health, a personal report will need to be written. This will follow the basic rules of an OH consultation with regard to consent and confidentiality.

Workplace visit report

An employee or group of employees or a manager may approach OH and request some advice or guidance about a work activity or environmental issue that is causing a potential health problem. These can range from insect infestations, lighting, heating or noise factors to workstation set-ups or use of equipment and ergonomic issues. Having established the 'facts', the OH nurse may wish to visit the site and see for him- or herself. This can often be done in liaison with other members of the OH team if available, e.g. physiotherapist, ergonomist, occupational hygienist if appropriate or with the safety adviser.

The outcome of any workplace visit is to report back to the individual(s) on the findings and, similarly to the management referral, offer some guidance on what might be put in place to alleviate the problem. Again these can only be recommendations; what is actually done is up to the management and budget considerations – what is reasonably practicable. However, the requirements for the report to be accurate, clear and concise are the same. The OH nurse is entitled to use judgement and professional opinion in recommending with awareness what is value for money (Figure 6.3).

An OH nurse may be required to submit a report to justify the expense of a new piece of equipment, e.g. the purchase of a newer model of a spirometer, or to bring

---

Date:
To: Line manager
                       HR manager
Re: Department or employee group

Hazards assessed

Health surveillance is a process of regular planned assessments of one or more aspects of a worker's health when a potential hazard to health has been identified by a risk assessment. This will have included the activities hazardous to health, the employees at risk and the measures taken to eliminate or reduce the risks. As a way of measuring the effectiveness of the controls, the group of employees can have various measurements, examinations, tests or questionnaires of their health undertaken. The results are then interpreted and employers advised on any actions required to eliminate or further control exposure. It may be necessary to redeploy affected workers if necessary. A health record is supplied for each individual in the target group. This report provides anonymised information and statistics on the group as a whole.

1. List of risks assessed based on the risk assessment
2. List of employees within the department/employee group (this should be updated annually prior to each yearly surveillance by management to ensure all at-risk employees are screened)
3. Number of assessments and did not attends
4. Percentage fit across group
5. Percentage unfit – if there is a pattern to this, a conclusion and advice will be offered to investigate possible causes for this, thus ensuring safe practices at work
6. Percentage of did not attends (management to be informed of individuals to follow up)

Complete a summary of the results for the group as a whole, with outcomes and feedback on the risk assessment and efficacy of current control measures. Individuals whose results indicate that they may be at current or future risk will be followed up and management will be informed so as to reassess the control measures. Health and safety recommendations may need to be discussed with health and safety adviser.

Signed: _____

Date: _____

Name and designation: _____

Figure 6.2 Template for a general report to management for health surveillance

in a new form of therapy, e.g. physiotherapy acupuncture, an increase in workforce by extra hours of OH admin time or a major project to justify a new build or a new contract. As with any business case, how big the report is will depend on the size of what is being asked for. If a report is requested by management then the content will need to follow the same pattern; the difference will be in the detail. There are plenty

---

Medical in Confidence*

Date:
To: Line manager
                             HR manager
Re: [Insert employee's name, staff no. (if available), job title and
                             department or an employee group details]
Workplace activity/
environmental factor: [Insert what the visit is primarily about]

[A brief description of the issue requiring an OH visit to the workplace]
[An outline of the work activity, with reference to work equipment, environment ergonomics, job
role, hours. Recommendations as to what needs to be improved to alleviate the health issues]
[Any health and safety issues – may need to liaise with safety adviser]

Signed: _____
Date: _____
Name and designation: _____

Figure 6.3 Template for a report to management following a workplace visit

*Only if a medical confidential issue is to be reported on.

of websites that give templates for business cases so these can be easily searched. The basic areas to cover are as follows:

- an executive summary
- background information
- strategic context
- proposal
- options and preferred option and why
- details of plan

- legal and financial implications
- funding
- timescale
- management arrangements
- resource implications
- key benefits and outcomes
- risk assessment
- conclusion.

Conclusion

Health assessment, supporting management with absence management and rehabilitation are now major parts of the OH nurse role. This aspect of OH practice is the cornerstone to maintaining an efficient and healthy workforce. Working in teams with a case management approach and considering the biopsychosocial aspects of the client are essential for good professional nursing practice.

References

1 Lewis J, Thornbory G (2010) *Employment Law and Occupational Health: A practical handbook*. Oxford: Wiley.
2 Kloss D (2010) *Occupational Health Law*. Oxford: Wiley.
3 Kloss D, Ballard J (2012) *Discrimination Law and Occupational Health Practice*. London: The At Work Partnership.
4 Thornbory G (1994) Health assessment in occupational health practice. MSc dissertation, unpublished.
5 Thornbory G (2013) Taking a history and making a functional assessment. *Occup Hlth* 65 (3): 27–29.
6 Palmer K, Cox R, Brown I (2007) *Fitness for Work: The medical aspects*, 4th edn. Faculty of Occupational Medicine. Oxford: Oxford University Press.
7 General Medical Council (2009) *Confidentiality: Guidance for Doctors*. GMC: London. Available online at: http://www.gmc-uk.org/Confidentiality_core_2009.pdf_27494212.pdf.
8 Pearson A, Vaughan B (1986) *Nursing Models for Practice*. London: Heinemann Nursing.
9 Bickley L (1999) *Bates Guide to Physical Examination and History Taking*, 7th edn. Philadelphia, PA: Lippincott.
10 Bjelland I, Dah I A A, Haug T T, Neckemann D (2002) The validity of the Hospital Anxiety and Depression Scale. An updated literature review. *J Psychosom Res* 52 (2): 69–77.
11 Hansard 7 Jan 2013 www.publications.parliament.uk/pa/cm201213/cmhansard/cm130117/detext/130117-0002.htm Columns 1053-1076 (accessed 28.04.13).
12 http://www.saunders-therapy.com/industrial.html.
13 https://www.roymatheson.com.
14 Templeman M (2006) *Wellbeing at Work: How to manage workplace wellness to boost your staff and business performance*. London: Institute of Directors. Available online at: http://www.director.co.uk/content/pdfs/wellbeing_guide.pdf (accessed 22.04.13).
15 Confederation of British Industry (2011) *Healthy Returns: Absence and workplace health survey*. Available online at: http://www.cbi.org.uk/media/955604/2011.05-healthy_returns_-_absence_and_workplace_health_survey_2011.pdf (accessed 22.04.13).

16 Chartered Institute of Personnel and Development (2012) *Absence Management: Annual survey*. Available online at: www.cipd.co.uk (accessed 22.04.13).

17 www.hse.gov.uk/statistics/index.htm.

18 http://www.cipd.co.uk/hr-resources/factsheets/absence-measurement-management. aspx (accessed 22.04.13).

19 Whitaker SC (2001) Management of sickness absence. *Occup Environ Med* 58 (6). Available online at: http://oem.bmj.com/content/58/6/420.full.pdf (accessed 27.04.11).

20 http://www.hse.gov.uk/sicknessabsence/index.htm (accessed 24.04.13).

21 Advisory Conciliation and Arbitration Service (2010) *Managing Attendance and Employee Turnover*. Available online at: www.acas.org.uk.

22 Chartered Institute of Personnel and Development (2006) *Absence Management 2: How do you develop an absence strategy?* Available online at: http://www.cipd.co.uk/binaries/absmanpractool2.pdf (accessed 27.04.11).

23 Black C (2008) *Working for a Healthier Tomorrow*. London: TSO. Available online at: http://www.dwp.gov.uk/docs/hwwb-working-for-a-healthier-tomorrow.pdf (accessed 08.07.13).

24 https://www.gov.uk/government/uploads/system/uploads/attachment_data/file/183335/fitnote-occupational-health-guide.pdf (accessed 24.04.13).

25 Silcox S (2004) Absence essentials: Return to work interviews. *Employment Rev* 810: 19–21. Available online at: http://icbr.net/pub/full_pdf/icbr.net-0202.12.pdf.

26 http://www.gmc-uk.org/guidance/ethical_guidance/confidentiality.asp (accessed 24.04.13).

27 Faculty of Occupational Medicine (2012) *Ethics Guidance for Occupational Health Practice*. Available online at: http://www.fom.ac.uk/publications-policy-guidance-and-consultations/publications/faculty-publications (accessed 24.04.13).

28 *Lyncock* v *Cereal Packing Ltd* (1988) 1 CR 670 EAT.

29 Case Management Society UK. Available online at: www.cmsuk.org (accessed 03.05.11).

30 Harrison T (2011) Leicester fit for work pilots. *Occup Hlth* 63 (5). Available online at: http://www.personneltoday.com/articles/01/09/2011/57684/how-effective-is-the-fit-for-work-service.htm#.Uds2LdLVCSo.

31 Waddell G, Burton AK (2004) *Concepts of Rehabilitation for the Management of Common Health Problems*. London: TSO

32 http://www.personneltoday.com/articles/18/07/2007/41581/government-sets-up-39vocational-rehabilitation39-taskforce.htm#.UXpgkrU3uPM.

33 Waddell G, Burton AK (2006) *Is Work Good for Your Health and Wellbeing?* London: TSO.

34 Vocational Rehabilitation Association (2007) *Standards of Practice*. London: VRA.

35 Farrell C, Nice K, Lewis J, Sainsbury R (2006) Experiences of the job retention and rehabilitation pilot. Research report 339. London: Department for Work and Pensions.

36 Hughes V (ed.) (2004) *Tolley's Guide to Employee Rehabilitation*. London: Lexis Nexis UK.

37 Kendall N, Burton AK (2009) *Tackling Musculoskeletal Problems: A guide for clinic and workplace*. London: TSO. Available online at: http://www.tsoshop.co.uk/bookstore. asp?FO=1299153 (accessed 03.05.11).

38 Nursing and Midwifery Council Code of Conduct. Available online at: http://www. nmc-uk.org.

39 Faculty of Occupational Medicine (2010) *Good Occupational Medical Practice*. London: Faculty of Occupational Medicine, p. 14.

40 Equality Act 2010. Available online at: https://www.gov.uk/rights-disabled-person/employment.

41 Carmel L (2012) Guidance on health case report writing. *Occup Health* 64: 27–29.

7 | Mental health at work

Anna Harrington

Learning objectives

After reading this chapter you will be able to:

- recognise the business and societal value of taking a strategic and integrated approach to mental health at work
- appreciate that the psychological environment within the workplace will have an effect on psychological wellbeing and employee performance
- recognise the key factors in the psychological environment that influence performance and health
- discuss the extent of mental ill health in the population at large and then the work population
- appreciate the effects of mental ill health on work performance and the workplace environment
- discuss the important aspects of assessing and giving a professional opinion about an individual with a mental health problem.

Why is mental health important?

This may come across as a question with an obvious answer, depending on your own attitude towards mental health. Talk to others around you to find out their thoughts and attitudes to mental health; it is likely to reveal that different attitudes do prevail. Some of these attitudes are damaging to mental health, which will be discussed later in stigma surrounding mental health.

A good starting point is to consider what effect mental health has on:

- individuals and families
- society at large
- workplaces.

Individuals and families

Good mental health allows people to lead lives that are personally fulfilling and enables the individual to contribute positively to others, therefore enhancing their lives. It can be said that the impact of one individual having good mental health is as great as the number of people on whom that person has a connection or relationship with. Common mental health problems are a frequently cited reason for loss of employment and sickness absence.[1,2,3] The loss of an income has a severe effect on the finances of a family. This brings with it associated tensions as forced change is needed in order to survive. Hopes and dreams are thwarted, leading to disappointment, frustration and despondency and the quality of life is diminished.[4] There is strong evidence to suggest the effects of worklessness on health increase mental and physical problems as well as mortality.[5] The effects within a family go beyond having the economic means to provide. Poverty is more than just the amount of money coming into the family. It is about the ability to seek opportunity, take that opportunity, to inspire and the creation of a stable environment. This is about the parent being able to create life chances for the child. The effects of poverty in families go beyond the childhood stage: they stretch into adulthood and pervade generations. There has been a suggestion that this also affects cognitive ability in future generations and therefore subsequent economic futures. Those children who are in families without a wage are more likely to suffer ill health.[6]

Society at large

It has been cited[4] that mental illness is the largest cause of disability and 13.8 per cent of England's health budget goes on mental health. That is the cost of treating the condition; it does not include the associated costs of care, welfare and reduced economic contribution. These are estimated to be £77 billion and are huge effects at a time when budgets need to be cut and measures put in place to rationalise spending. The majority of mental illness is in the common mental ill-health category. However, it should not go unrecognised that mental illness often does not exist in isolation but is frequently accompanied by significant physical health problems. These physical health problems can be the result of the mental health problem or associated medication or be a causative factor in mental ill health. As mentioned in the previous section, the effects of mental health are largely felt by the individual and their families. Estimates of this consider loss of earnings, thwarted potential and quality of life. Figures suggest that 30 per cent of the costs are assigned to society and 70 per cent to the individual.[7]

Mental ill health can start early, from the age of 14, and continue on into old age. It is reported that childhood mental ill health is growing. The most common type of mental ill health in children is anxiety and/or depression. Many continue to have these problems into adulthood. Dementia is said to be an issue that will grow and have an increasing impact on society, individuals and families.[8] Poor mental health is associated with low achievement, increase in health risk behaviours, social exclusion and criminality. Each of these brings significant damage to society in the form of affecting social cohesion and communities. It is right to say that raising mental health issues in society brings a reduction in antisocial behaviour disorders, criminality, increased life expectancy, increased skills and therefore contribution to society.[9] Mental ill health not just affects society due to the draw on public resources but it limits the potential of society to be thriving and economically contributing to the country.[7] In the Department of Health strategy,[9] communities which are thriving and supportive improve the well-being and mental health of those connected with it. The document also states that depression in the older population is growing and that 25 per cent of older people have depression; life expectancy is increasing, putting pressure on the public purse and pensions. The result of all this is that people need to delay the age of retirement. It has therefore become increasingly important for good working health to be extended into older age.

Workplaces

It has been estimated that at any one time one in six workers will have a mental health problem. This figure changes to one in five if drug and alcohol problems are included.[10] Mental ill health continues to be in the top five reasons for absence. When breaking down this figure to look at long-term absence, mental ill health is the top figure that is reported. Figures to identify the costs of absence currently are estimated at £600 per employee per year.[11] Surveys on the impact of health at work suggest that, while the total absence figure is dropping, there is an impact on an individual's ability to work at a level that is acceptable to the employer. This is known as presenteeism, where the individual is physically at work, but not fully engaged and productive. It is thought that, as employment status is more precarious, individuals will be at work and are less likely to take time off. Whilst it could be considered more beneficial to have an employee at work than off, this needs to be set against the consequence of poor performance.[12] How does it affect team morale and cohesiveness? What about effects on customer relations? Mental ill health is also known to have a detrimental effect on decision making and concentration. It has been estimated that the costs of presenteeism are one and a half times the costs of absence.[10] However, businesses are often not aware of these facts and many fail to consider that the problem is one that affects them.[10] Yet how can mental health not affect them, when the number of adults in the population who have a mental health problem is significant? In addition, this is not a situation that will disappear overnight, as distressingly the number of children who are experiencing mental health problems is also on the rise; after all, the children are the future workforce. It therefore stands to reason that businesses need help to recognise the issue, and to become more able to prevent problems and assist in resolving or reducing the impact. There are a number of well-known, large, high-performing businesses that are significantly investing in initiatives such as wellbeing. These businesses have also demonstrated huge returns on investment for initiatives which have ranged from recruitment methods and raising awareness to the provision of suitable support.[13] The majority of workers are not employed in these businesses; most work in the small to medium-sized sector. Therefore the majority of the working-age population and businesses are not having issues relating to work and mental health being addressed. Work is good for health – that is a generally agreed statement that came from the Waddell and Burton study, *Is Work Good for Your Health?*,[5] but the detail of this needs to be agreed – what is good work?

Definitions

Terms such as health, mental health and wellbeing are frequently used. There is much overlap between the definitions of mental health and wellbeing.

Mental health

> Mental health is defined as a state of well-being in which every individual realizes his or her own potential, can cope with the normal stresses of life, can work productively and fruitfully, and is able to make a contribution to her or his community.[14]

Wellbeing

The World Health Organization aligns wellbeing with mental health; other sources refer to it as being contented, healthy or successful. The most occupationally significant and clear definition relates to mental health:

> *Mental/psychological wellbeing* is a dynamic state in which the individual is able to develop their potential, work productively and creatively, build strong and positive relationships with others and contribute to their community. It is enhanced when an individual is able to fulfil their personal and social goals and achieve a sense of purpose in society.[8]

Wellbeing can be explained as having two aspects: the first is the immediate happiness, pleasure effects (hedonic), which are important to balance the negative, more difficult impacts of day-to-day living. The other aspect is about self-actualisation and fulfilment (eudaimonic).[15] This side of wellbeing brings with it encountering difficult, challenging but desired experiences. Desired because usually they contribute to a longer-term goal; the satisfactory feeling of working towards a greater purpose can feed fulfilment. The debate about different types of happiness that may contribute to wellbeing remains open.[15] The Foresight report[8] proposed five ways to wellbeing:

1. Connect with others. Identify people and relationships in your life that have influence, and build stronger relationships with these people.
2. Be active. Activity positively impacts physical, cognitive and emotional health.
3. Take notice. Take the time and opportunity to notice properly and consider positively the beauty and good things in your life.
4. Keep learning: this feeds self-worth and belief (self-esteem).
5. Give.

Mental capital

This encompasses individuals' cognitive and emotional resources. It includes their cognitive ability, how flexible and efficient they are at learning and their 'emotional intelligence', such as their social skills and resilience in the face of stress. It therefore conditions how well an individual is able to contribute effectively to society, and also to experience a high personal quality of life.[8]

Mental capital has obvious links and importance to the occupational setting.

In this chapter the terms mental health and wellbeing will be used interchangeably.

Stigma and discrimination

Stigma is felt by many who have a mental illness. According to Thornicroft,[16] this is not just a problem in the UK, but is experienced around the world by those who have a mental health problem. It affects many life domains: work, family, healthcare system, personal relationships, financial and insurance needs. Studies have shown common experiences, such as:

- most people would rather not be friends with families of a relative who has a mental illness
- abuse from neighbours: this can be verbal, or offensive property damage, marking out the individual, so highlighting the stigma
- denied employment
- made redundant
- shame from themselves and blame from others
- avoiding involvement in the community
- avoiding discussing care needs.

Stigma is an important issue that needs to be considered in the workplace and addressed. It is a sign or mark that identifies the wearer as being different. Historically it is associated as a physical mark deliberately made to warn others to avoid the person marked out. It has also been associated with physical illness, such as leprosy, again associated with fear – fear of disease transmission. It can be said to be a sign or mark, either physical or psychological, that identifies the person as being different from society's expected and accepted norms. The stigmatisation of an individual or group guides others to deploy actions and behaviours to keep them from being affected by the difference which has marked the other person out. It is said to have a number of different components:

- labelling – in which the difference is noted and recognised as being significant
- stereotyping – the connection of that difference to something that is undesirable. The undesirable could be behaviour, a way of being or linking to status, achievement and potential
- separating – the exclusion and segregation of those with stigma from those without

- status loss and discrimination – the individual or group's life is given less value than unaffected others. Barriers are presented which prevent the individual or group from fully participating in society.

It can also be thought of as having a number of fundamentals underlying the components:[17,18]

- ignorance and myths
- prejudice and negative attitudes
- discriminating behaviour.

These actions and behaviours then affect the way affected individuals live their life. Frequently social networks of those with a mental health problem will be small and often limited to those who have a similar experience. This is especially so with sufferers of severe mental health illness. People with mental ill health will avoid situations where discrimination and exclusion are likely to be experienced, so will decide not to apply for a job because of presumed reactions and behaviours. Karsay[19] states that this is self-limiting behaviour, brought about by presumed discrimination, which is not always borne out. Therefore individuals avoid putting themselves in that situation and this results in a vicious circle, with opportunities for development and life enhancement being limited by a loss of faith, trust and confidence.

Worryingly, it has also been said to affect the level of care and treatment from healthcare services.[16] It is recognised that people with a mental health problem have shorter lives than those without.

Work enhances social acceptance and social status and can build confidence and improve socialisation.[5] However, obstacles are found at every stage of the employment process. Barriers are placed at the point of diagnosis or treatment, with healthcare staff suggesting their ability to work is severely affected.[17] The declaration of a mental ill health problem at job application stage reduces the chances of employment when set against a physical problem.[18] Those with a mental health problem are at double the risk of losing their job when compared to those without a mental health problem. The comparator includes people with a physical health problem. In employment commonly the declaration of a mental health problem is reserved until trust and confidence have been built up. However even at that stage the declaration of disclosure still brings with it risks of being excluded and rejected.[17] These consequences bear out the figures associated with the employment of disabled people, according to Thornicroft. Sixty-five per cent of people with a physical health problem are employed, 50 per cent with a common mental health problem are employed and only 20 per cent with a severe mental health problem are employed.[17]

This discrimination has been evident at the heart of British bureaucracy. The Mental Health Act 1983 prevented members of parliament from undertaking their parliamentary work if they have been detained under the Act. However, all these barriers were removed by the Mental Health (Discrimination) Act 2013. According to Kloss and Ballard,[20] the Equality Act 2010 defines a disabling mental impairment as a protected characteristic. It must be long-term (12 months or more) and substantially interfere with normal day-to-day activities. It does not need to be a clinically well-recognised mental illness. The employer has a duty to avoid both direct and indirect discrimination and to make reasonable adjustments for those with a disability. Direct discrimination is making an automatic assumption, for example, that because an employee has a mental illness he or she will be incapable of taking a post with greater responsibility, and is always unlawful.

However this requires businesses to be aware of the legislation and how attitudes can be unnoticed and unrecognised and yet have a significant limiting effect on an individual. Rethink is a charity that aims to challenge and change attitudes about mental ill health. They work together with the mental health charity Mind to develop and run a government-funded programme.[21]

Organisation culture, engagement and wellbeing

Individual human beings do not thrive or survive well on their own. Humans need to live with others in order to have a chance of fulfilment and happiness. This survival need pushes people together in groups and communities. A workplace is a group of people – at its best a thriving community, at its worst a group of individuals. Work can be good for health and this includes mental wellbeing,[5] but it has to be the right type of work for this to be actualised. Work needs to be meaningful and to be managed well not just to avoid the situations and psychological/social environments which impinge on wellbeing but also to grasp opportunities that promote wellbeing. The promotion of wellbeing has the potential to bring with it an employee who is more engaged.[22]

Employee engagement

This is really a human resources (HR) issue rather an occupational health (OH) issue. However it must be remembered that OH is as much about the promotion of health as it is about the prevention of ill health – see Chapter 1. The definition of employee engagement by Clarke and Macleod[23] will serve to illuminate why OH and HR issues are included in this chapter: 'a workplace approach designed to ensure that employees are committed to their organisation's goals and values, motivated to contribute to organisational success, and are able at the same time to enhance their own sense of well-being.'

As you can see from this definition, the role of engagement is twofold – to feed the antecedents which allow for some business success, i.e. commitment to organisation goals and values but also to enhance individual life experience through the contribution to wellbeing. True, full engagement is through the inclusion of the emotional aspects of the individual in order to contribute to wellbeing. These factors are not to be excluded; they are important. Not all definitions of engagement will go this far to include the wellbeing experiences[24] and so consequently not all workplaces will automatically recognise that considering employee health to this level will assist individuals to work better as teams, go beyond the expected to achieve customer satisfaction and offer up voluntarily innovations and ideas. This in turn will lead to increased profits, a workplace that is buzzing, where recruitment costs are low due to low employee turnover and a reputation that attracts high-calibre potential employees.[24]

Occuptional health and employee engagement

A major role of OH is to contribute to business success. Through assisting the business in devising and implementing strategies to enhance employee wellbeing, OH aims to achieve both improved health and wellbeing for employees as well as better business for the company. With the difficult economic situation in the world, and particularly the UK, the working situation is changing. Businesses are exploring how the best can really be encouraged from each and every worker.[24] For this to happen employee wellbeing needs to be a serious consideration. According to Business in the Community,[25] businesses with high levels of employee wellbeing are more likely to have high engagement and are the most profitable. Researchers have found that workers who are unhappy use behaviours which result in their unhappiness being spread to others. In contrast others have found that happy workers are able to see opportunities, be more helpful to coworkers and are more confident.[25] Employees with high levels of wellbeing are less likely to see ambiguous events as threatening. Workplace change brings with it varying degrees of ambiguity as problems are worked through and understood, and solutions found and implemented. A business where the employees have high levels of wellbeing is less likely to experience some of the fallout from change such as increased anxiety and stress levels in employees. Critical feedback is more likely to be felt by employees with low levels of wellbeing. People with lower levels of wellbeing are more likely to use problematic interpersonal behaviours, therefore affecting others in the workplace.[24] High levels of wellbeing release creativity, positivity towards challenges, zest for life, problem-solving skills and greater ability to connect socially and influence.

What business would not want to see high wellbeing and engagement attributes exhibited by its employees?

How can this be achieved in the workplace?

It has been said that workplaces that are able to provide meaningful and challenging, but manageable, tasks are likely to encourage positive emotional states such as joy, energy, pleasure and more fulfilment effects such as growth. Some aspects of culture which are said to have an impact on wellbeing, according to TowersPerrin,[26] can be seen in Box 7.1.

Box 7.1 TowersPerrin aspects of culture which affect wellbeing

- Physical environment
- Leadership effectiveness
- Working relationships
- Sense of competency
- Aspirations and need for personal growth
- Views on access and fairness of performance
- Work–life balance
- Work overload
- Organisation commitment
- Job security
- Control/autonomy
- Resources and communications
- Pay and benefits
- Job satisfaction
- Sense of purpose
- Engagement
- Positive psychological wellbeing, physical and psychological health

Source: TowersPerrin (2006) *Employee Wellbeing: Taking engagement and performance to the next level*. Available online at: www.bitc.org.uk (accessed 23.11.12).

The power of leaders and influencers

An organisational culture is created by those in the organisation; as you go higher up the organisation the need for this to be a positive influence increases.[27] The 2010 Confederation of British Industry/Pfizer study[28] into absence and workplace health found that focusing on workplace culture had the same level of impact on absence as closer absence management. The group which has the biggest impact on culture, wellbeing and engagement is those with authority such as line managers and those who take the lead in the organisation. The leaders in the organisation have the influence to affect employee wellbeing, and associated productivity and attachment to the organisation.[29] The limelight needs first to be directed towards the key leaders and boards of organisations. According to Mowbray,[30] this is currently unlikely to be a primary focus for this group as ways of squeezing more from less have taken priority during the economic downturn. An alternative priority, of placing the workforce at the centre of the organisation strategy, is argued as being the most efficient way of creating a high-performing organisation. The theory is that if the workforce feels well and happy, then the processes required in making a profitable business will occur naturally. This will happen with little need for the coercive behaviour that would impact negatively on wellbeing.[30] It also creates organisational freedom, as the need for

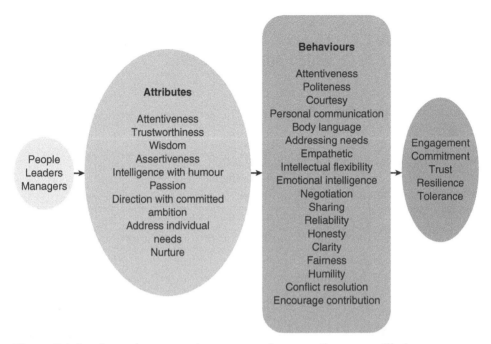

Figure 7.1 Leader and manager demeanours that contribute to wellbeing

With kind permission from Derek Mowbray (2007) Attributes and behaviours (diagram).

rules, monitoring and restriction becomes less,[31] allowing managers to discover who their employees are and what is important to them. Individuals will want to give to the team and the organisation as the rewards feed their need for fulfilment and personal satisfaction. It is a symbiotic and reciprocal relationship. The reason that this occurs is because the workforce will feel valued: they will recognise that their interests are of primary importance to the organisation and that they will be given recognition which is meaningful to them.

Organisations with engaged staff have clear evidence of trust, mutual respect and fairness; promises are understood and fulfilled. Figure 7.1 shows the types of manager and leader demeanours which will contribute positively to wellbeing.

Behaviour which leads to a healthy sense of wellbeing should be ingrained within the company when considering the organisation culture. It should also be explicit so expectations are clear. Mowbray[31] suggests that having a standard of behaviour is a useful idea. Once the culture has been set it is necessary to assist those who are given positions of power, such as the managers, in considering their own behaviours and adapting accordingly. The Health and Safety Executive (HSE) has produced a behavioural competency tool which can be used to assess four behaviour areas which, if used, contribute to controlling and preventing stress in others.[32]

Role and value of occupational health

The position of the OH nurse is unique in that it allows for the gathering of factors which may be affecting the employee's ability to work; this includes personal as well as work factors. Therefore it could be suggested that the role of OH is to illuminate to the board regarding the factors that are affecting wellbeing and performance[33] as the relevant data is collected routinely in the day-to-day tasks of an OH adviser (OH nurse). For example, when conducting surveillance for hand–arm vibration, the OH nurse will be discussing with the employee the workplace factors that are causing concern. A large part of the work of an OH nurse is to see people with health-related performance issues who have been referred by management. The very heart of this consultation process is the exploration of the workplace from the employee perspective. This will include factors that are impinging on wellbeing.

Work is good for one's health, according to Waddell and Burton,[5] but it has to be the right type of work. Hopefully above is an exploration of the right type of work from a mental health/psychological wellbeing perspective. Now we will explore some of the psychological problems that may occur when the employee regards the work as unsatisfactory.

Stress

For some years it has been noted that stress-related problems are affecting individuals and business. The 2012 and 2011 Chartered Institute of Personnel Development (CIPD) absence surveys[11] place stress in the top four reasons for causing sickness absence. This remains the same for public-sector, private-sector, manual or non-manual workers. However rates are higher in the public and not-for-profit sectors. These figures match those from the HSE,[34] which state that 'occupations that report the highest rates of total cases of work-related stress (three-year average) were health professionals (in particular nurses), teaching and educational professionals, and caring personal services (in particular welfare and housing associate professionals)'. These statistics are gathered from the Labour Force Survey and revealed that 40 per cent of cases were stress. This survey is conducted by the Office for National Statistics on a quarterly basis. According to this survey, in 2011–2012 10.4 million working days were lost to stress.[26]

What is stress?

There are a number of definitions of stress. The HSE states that it is the result of little attention being paid to work design, work organisation and management and that it leaves the individual feeling unable to cope.[35] Another definition is 'the pattern of specific and nonspecific responses an organism makes to stimulus events that disturb its equilibrium and tax or exceed its ability to cope.'[36] The International Stress Management Association[37] states: 'stress manifests as a physical, psychological or social dysfunction resulting in individuals feeling unable to bridge the gap with the requirements or expectations placed upon them.' All these definitions identify two issues – the feeling of individuals not being able to manage and the nature of the requirements that are being made of them. This definition is the one that may be regarded as the most all-encompassing:

a pattern of emotional, cognitive, behavioural and physiological reactions to adverse and noxious aspects of work content, work organisation and work environment. It is a state characterised by high levels of arousal and distress and often by feelings of not coping.[38]

The definition details that it is a total-body response to an external stimuli. It also suggests that the feeling of not coping is a consequence of the stimuli, similar to the other definitions. This then should give guidance as to how it can be prevented, that is, to consider the character and features of the work. However, first let's explore what happens and the signs and symptoms.

Stress: biological components

The very complicated biological mechanisms associated with stress were described in a seminal piece of work by Hans Selye.[39] Since then, the main principles of his discovery have been expanded upon. One of his frustrations was that the term stress came to be linked with something distressing, forgetting about the positive stress that is also experienced. To assist in giving clarity to this definition Selye also coined the term eustress, meaning stress that is positive to the individual. He described an agent later known as a stressor causing the release of corticotrophic hormone-releasing factor from within the brain and working in the brain to release adrenocorticotrophic hormone. This goes into the general blood circulation and causes the release of corticoids, such as glucocorticoid to create energy for the expected reactions. It is thought that corticoids also suppress the immune system and inflammatory responses. Catecholamines are also released – adrenaline, which speeds up the heart rate, raises blood pressure and accelerates blood coagulation. There is also thought to be a biofeedback mechanism. These acute stress responses are to prepare the body for a survival reaction, usually a physical response. If the stressor is diminished or disappears then the individual will return to normal homeostasis; however this response starts to cause real issues when it is continued over a long period of time.

Signs and symptoms

The biological mechanisms and signs and symptoms of stress can be seen in Box 7.2.

Workplace pressure management

To prevent stress psychological pressure levels need to be managed in the workplace. The HSE and CIPD have devised a number of frameworks and tools to be used to ensure pressure is kept at performance-enhancing and low risk to health levels.[33] The HSE recommends that stress is assessed using the five-step risk assessment process (see Figure 5.5 in Chapter 5) and that the six domains are considered in the risk assessment. These domains have been defined after the collation of extensive research studies suggesting the main causes of stress. They are as follows:

Box 7.2 The biological mechanisms, signs and symptoms of stress

Increased heart rate
Increased blood pressure
More susceptible to some infections
Sweating
Skin complaints such as eczema
Suppression of appetite/nausea/butterflies
Muscle tension and increased complaints of musculoskeletal problems
Reproductive problems

Behavioural/mood effects

Anxiety
Depression
More emotional
Changes in behaviour
Increased irritability

Source: Cohen S, Frank E, Doyle WJ, Skoner DP, Rabin BS, Gwaltney JM (1998) Types of stressors that increase the susceptibility to the common cold in healthy adults. *Hlth Psychol* 17 (3): 214–223.

- Demands – this includes issues such as workload, work patterns and the work environment.
- Control – how much say individuals have in the way they do their work.
- Support – this includes the encouragement, sponsorship and resources provided by the organisation, line management and colleagues.
- Relationships – this includes promoting positive working to avoid conflict and dealing with unacceptable behaviour.
- Role – whether people understand their role within the organisation and whether the organisation ensures that they do not have conflicting roles.
- Change – how organisational change (large or small) is managed and communicated in the organisation.

Mental health disorders

Mental health disorders cover a range of affective states and derangements of thoughts and perceptions. These can affect abilities on all levels, for example the ability to complete basic human functions and to process information. Frequently an individual with a mental health disorder will also have a physical health condition.[9] In addition it is

Table 7.1 Prevalence rates for psychiatric morbidity

Disorder	Prevalence rate 2007
Reported suicidal thoughts	16.7%
Common mental health disorder	15.1%
ADHD	8.2%
Suicidal attempts	5.6%
Self-harm	4.9%
PTSD	3%
Psychosis	0.4%
ASPD	0.3%
BPD	0.4%

ADHD, attention deficit hyperactivity disorder; PTSD, posttraumatic stress disorder; ASPD, antisocial personality disorder; BPD, borderline personality disorder.

not uncommon for an individual to have two or more psychiatric disorders.[40] A psychiatric disorder may be diagnosed using the *Diagnostic Statistical Manual of Mental Disorders* – otherwise known as DSM-IV. This tome is presented by the American Psychiatric Association. There is also the *International Classification of Diseases-10* (ICD-10), produced by the World Health Organization (Table 7.1) which contains the most recent prevalence rates for psychiatric morbidity.

Common mental health disorders (CMD) include anxiety, depression and a mixture of the two.[41] They cause distress and disrupt function but do not result in distorted thinking and insight. Of those who presented with a CMD in this survey, more than half were a mix between anxiety and depression. Of the 15 per cent, 24 per cent were receiving treatment (mainly medication), which leaves 76 per cent who were not receiving treatment. This is obviously alarming when considering the potential effects of these disorders on an individual's ability to perform work tasks up to a required standard.

Psychoses are disorders that affect cognitive ability and perceptions of reality. The main types are schizophrenia and affective psychosis (bipolar, for example).[41] Eighty per cent of those who were identified in this study were receiving treatment, either medication and/or counselling. The most significant issue with people diagnosed with these disorders is adherence to treatment. The medication has side-effects that some find difficult to tolerate and their positive effects can result in individuals believing that they no longer require them.

Here we will focus on the CMD and suicidal thoughts, as these are the ones that are most likely to be experienced in the workplace according to the survey.

Common mental health disorders and the OH nurse consultation

Certain associations can be connected with CMD and it is important for the OH nurse to be aware of these. During a consultation these should be explored. Through exploration an understanding of causative factors will be gained and therefore appropriate advice and signposting can be given. However, with some of the associations it is not

Table 7.2 Associations and some effects of common mental health disorders

Associations

- Debt and financial problems
- Gender
- Work stress
- Social isolation
- Poor housing
- Negative life events
- Poor physical health
- Family history of depression
- Poor interpersonal and family relationships
- Partner in poor health
- Problems with alcohol
- Marital status
- Educational attainment

Somatic symptoms

- Fatigue
- Unable to find pleasure in life
- Loss of interest in things
- Irritability
- Problems with concentration, decision making and memory
- Loss of confidence
- Agitation
- Poor sleep
- Unable to complete daily tasks
- Worry
- Compulsions
- Obsessions

Source: Lindsey J, Baillon S, Brugha T *et al.* (2006) Worry content across a life span: an analysis of 160 74 year old participants in the British National Survey of Psychiatric Morbidity 2000. *Psychol Med* 36 (11): 1625–1633.

clear whether they are a result of the illness or if the illness caused them, for example, debt and financial problems[41] (Table 7.2).

The National Institute for Health and Clinical Excellence (NICE) guides clinicians to use the ICD-10[42] or DSM-IV[43] to formulate a diagnosis. However this is not the role of the OH nurse, although one needs to be aware of symptoms, signs, severity and the effects of these on function and causes in order to be able to advise the employer and employee appropriately on the best way forward in terms of work. The other reason for being aware of the symptoms is that many people often do not access a diagnosis and treatment for CMD.[44] The OH nurse may be able to guide the employee to seek advice and treatment from the general practitioner or other appropriate body (such as Improving Access to Psychological Treatment service).

From the list of symptoms it should be evident that the impact on work ability could be significant. The OH nurse will need to understand the level of significance/impact for the individual and his or her work.

Work effects of mental ill health

Mental health problems can affect the following:

- Concentration and attention: This can be the result of medication or the illness itself, causing the individual to be occupied with internal mental thoughts and worries. Quick and simple tests such as 'serial 7s' can be used to get an understanding of the level of effect[45] or simply asking individuals to give a percentage score of how they feel their concentration level is when compared to their norm. This latter method of assessment is obviously relying on individuals having the appropriate level of self-awareness.

- Impaired motor skills: Some drugs, such as selective serotonin reuptake inhibitors, used to treat mental ill health, can result in the person feeling motionless or controlling motion. In addition the disorder itself may result in these problems.[46]
- Impaired communication and social skills:[45] This can be the result of problems associated with the illness such as isolation, low self-confidence and poor self-esteem.

OH assessment

The purpose of an OH assessment is usually about offering advice and recommendations to the individual and employer, about adaptations that may be needed to enable the individual to perform the required tasks.[34] It is possible that the OH nurse will be asked to give an opinion about performance standards and limitations of the individual. This can be one of the most challenging tasks within OH, as there is often not a set standard against which individuals can be measured.[44] As mental health problems may be undiagnosed the OH nurse should be mindful of this when assessing those who may not be presenting with a mental health problem. For depression two questions can be asked:

1. During the last month, have you often been bothered by feeling down, depressed or hopeless?
2. During the last month, have you often been bothered by having little interest or pleasure in doing things?[31]

In addition mental illness brings with it a degree of unpredictability, partly due to differing individual responses to treatment. It is therefore essential that the individual's responses and symptoms are placed at the centre of the consultation. Inquiries into the usual past medical history and history of presenting condition will be made during the consultation and certain other domains will need to be explored with the individual. These include fluctuating conditions relating to the person such as concentration, memory, motivation, lifestyle (exercise, diet, including drugs and alcohol, personal relationships, home stresses and strains) and previous employment history.[34] The use of standardised assessment tools such as the Hospital Anxiety Depression Scale can be useful to provide further data about the type and severity of the disorder.[43] They can also be used as a benchmark against which future assessments can be made. It may be necessary for the OH nurse to assess how the illness or disease is affecting functional ability. This varies greatly as factors such as coping mechanisms, adaptive skills and motivation all come into play. It has also been suggested that the OH service should be more involved in suicide prevention through making enquiries of individuals who are in 'at-risk' groups.[45] High-risk groups include:

- young and middle-aged men
- people in the care of mental health services
- people with a history of self-harm
- people in contact with the criminal justice system
- specific occupational groups – nurses, doctors, veterinary workers, farmers, agricultural workers.[47]

A professional judgement is made by gathering information about current fitness for work, future fitness for work and adaptations. It is also at this stage that the OH nurse needs to consider the applicability of the Equality Act.

Workplace factors

In addition particular workplace factors need to be examined such as the level of pressure and strain. This can be done using the HSE stress management standards, or considering styles of management through the CIPD/HSE/Investors in People behavioural competency framework.[48] Other considerations include flexible working opportunities, shift work and attitude to work. All these need to be considered alongside the organisation culture and the individual's perceptions/interpretations of the situation.

Treatment

Treatment is the responsibility of the individual's general practitioner or hospital consultant. However, the OH nurse needs to be aware of the recommended treatment methods and responses. In formulating a judgement the OH nurse will need to assess the prescribed treatments being used. On the advice of an occupational physician, employers may choose to offer one of the recommended treatments following guidance from NICE. Treatments such as computerised cognitive behavioural therapy have been shown to have positive business outcomes such as reduced time off sick.[49]

Return to work

Returning to work for an individual who has been absent with a mental health problem can seem frightening and daunting. This may also be a barrier to returning to work, especially if it relates to the stigma associated with mental ill health, loss of confidence and self-belief. It could also relate to other factors such as loss of mental and physical stamina and difficulties at certain times of the day such as mornings. One of the biggest barriers is the perception of managers and individuals that a full recovery needs to be made before a return to work is attempted. However, appropriate work can be part of the recovery/rehabilitation phase. This has the advantage to the employer of having the individual back doing some work and reduces the amount of sick time. Rehabilitation needs to be carefully managed and the organisation culture will have a large part to play in the success of this. It is advisable that the OH nurse is fully involved with the employee in devising a return-to-work plan and communicating/negotiating this with the employer. It is also useful to involve the community mental health team by obtaining information from them about progress in treatment, outcomes and opinions on work factors[46] with the employee's written consent.

Case study 7.1

An experienced social worker was off work for 4 months with an anxiety disorder. She felt she wanted to start back doing some work because she was frustrated and bored at home. She was coming to the end of her cognitive behavioural therapy sessions, which she said had assisted her in identifying her thought patterns which were often destructive and she had developed skills to challenge these thoughts. She had also completed a course of mindfulness which had taught her relaxation techniques. Her fears about work were that as she is an experienced member of the team she would be expected to jump straight back into her role.

- How would an OH nurse help with her return to work?

First, the OH nurse will need to undertake a full assessment of the situation and form a judgement of the social worker's readiness to start back to work. As well as the usual questions related to past medical history (where relevant), medication and treatment, social history, present lifestyle (diet, exercise, drugs and alcohol, sleep), there are a few questions that need to be asked regarding the current problem:

- Were there any workplace issues which contributed to the problem?
- What are her current abilities?
- What are her current limitations?
- What are her barriers to work (biopsychosocial)?
- What adjustments does she feel would address limitations and barriers?
- What length of time would these adjustments need to be in place for?
- What sort of contact has she had with the workplace?

If the OH nurse believes that a return to work is timely the next stage of the conversation needs to focus on what, if any, adaptations can be suggested to the social worker's manager (Box 7.3). These suggested adjustments can be useful for many mental health problems. A significant aspect of this is that individuals feel in control, fully involved, able to say no and to offer up adjustments which they feel would be useful.

Box 7.3 Examples of adaptations/adjustments

Emotional/confidence

Allowance/permission to take time out to use practised relaxation techniques

Regular positive feedback

Daily scheduled work tasks identified clearly

Standards clearly communicated

Clarity over medium- and longer-term plans/goals

Open and honest communication between all parties

Provide a buddy in whom she has trust

Mentor to allow for necessary relearning of job

Concentration

Keep distractions to a minimum – auditory and visual

Break up bigger pieces of work into smaller tasks

Encourage focus on one task at a time

Have dedicated short concentration periods and then microbreaks, for example, 20 minutes' concentration, 2 minutes away

Take formal breaks away from the work environment, ideally outside

Use natural daylight to light work space

Memory

Allow the use of memory aids such as taping discussions about work tasks, minute/note taking

Provide written instructions

Regular reviews of work

Colour-code work into priority order – red, amber and green

Use tick charts and lists

Fatigue/mental stamina

Allow for a phased return to fulltime/contracted hours. For example, start on half of the contracted hours and build up by 1–2 hours per week

Allow for greater time to complete tasks

Flexi-working

Work from home

(continued)

(continued)

Take formal breaks away from the work area, ideally outside, and use micro-breaks from tasks

Relationships

Encourage an informal get-together between the individual, line manager and other person from the workplace whom the person trusts and has a bond with

Encourage open, honest and respectful communications

Agree about how colleagues will be involved and informed about the return to work

Source: Adapted from http://askjan.org/media/Psychiatric.html (accessed 16.4.13).

Advanced decisions

An advanced statement is usually connected with a serious mental illness and details individuals' wishes with regard to their care when they themselves are incapable of making rational judgements. The legal rules are found in the Mental Capacity Act 2005. Although not needing to be detailing treatment, the principles of setting out measures to enable safety and care of the individual are of benefit in the workplace; they can assist open communication and appropriate and fair management of the work and roles which the individual is required to do but may temporarily be unable to perform due to acute exacerbation. It is about setting out agreements about the way the individual and organisation decide on how to enable work to continue safely for the individual and the organisation. An advanced statement can bring a level of psychological security to the individual and the organisation. It can include the following details:[50]

- who to contact if an acute episode of illness occurs whilst at work
- what early signs and symptoms are noticeable and suggest deterioration in health
- if any of these are identified, how and by whom the individual should be approached
- what can be done at work to prevent further deterioration
- where the advanced statement is to be stored and who has access to it.

Conclusion

Mental health at work is a broad subject. Good mental health and wellbeing have the potential to drive a business forward. Poor mental health and wellbeing will have rippling effects that are costly financially as well as detrimental to the quality of life of all who are touched by them. OH contributes positively in the advancement of good workplace mental health by channelling it through the wellbeing and engagement agendas. It is constraining to business development to have a focus on only one aspect of mental health such as mental ill health. Adopting a strategic and integrated blueprint to workplace mental health will allow for it to release the potential of all employees and develop sound business.

References

1 www.jrf.org.uk/publications/child-poverty-and-its-consquences (accessed 9.1.12).
2 Black C (2008) *Working for a Healthier Tomorrow*. London: TSO. Available online at: http://www.dwp.gov.uk/docs/hwwb-working-for-a-healthier-tomorrow.pdf (accessed 5.4.13).
3 McManus S, Mowlam A, Dorsett R *et al.* (2012) *Mental Health in Context: The National Study of work-search and wellbeing*. Research report 810. DWP. Available online at: http://research.dwp.gov.uk/asd/asd5/rports2011-2012/rrep810.pdf (accessed 5.4.13).
4 National Mental Health Development Unit DH. *Fact File 3: The cost of mental ill health*. Available online at: http://www.nmhdu.org.uk/silo/files/nmhdu-factfile-3.pdf (accessed 5.3.13).
5 Waddell G, Burton AK (2006) *Is Work Good for Your Health?* Norwich: TSO. Available online at: http://www.dwp.gov.uk/docs/hwwb-is-work-good-for-you.pdf (accessed 14.7.13).
6 DWP and Department of Education (2011) *A New Approach to Child Poverty: Tackling the causes of disadvantaged and transforming lives*. London: TSO. Available online at: https://www.education.gov.uk/publications/eOrderingDownload/CM-8061.pdf (accessed 5.4.13).
7 Sainsbury's Centre for Mental Health (2003) *The Economic and Social Costs of Mental Illness*. Policy paper 3. Available online at: http://www.centreformentalhealth.org.uk/pdfs/costs_of_mental_illness_policy_paper_3.pdf (accessed 5.4.13).
8 Foresight (2008) *Mental Capital and Wellbeing Project. Final Report*. London: The Government Office for Science. Available online at: http://www.bis.gov.uk/assets/biscore/corporate/migratedD/ec_group/116-08-FO_b (accessed 5.4.13).
9 Department of Health (2003) *No Health Without Mental Health: A cross-government mental health outcomes strategy for people of all ages*. Available online at: http://www.iapt.nhs.uk/silo/files/no-health-without-mental-health.pdf (accessed 5.4.13).
10 Sainsbury Centre for Mental Health (2007) *Mental Health at Work: Developing the business case*. Policy 8. Available online at: http://www.centreformentalhealth.org.uk/pdfs/mental_health_at_work.pdf (accessed 5.4.13).
11 Chartered Institute of Personnel Development and Simply Health (2012) *Absence Management Annual Survey Report*. Available online at: https://www.simplyhealth.co.uk/shcore/sh/content/pdfs/cipd_survey_2012.pdf (accessed 5.4.13).
12 The Work Foundation (2009) *Why Do Employees Come to Work When Ill? An investigation into sickness presence in the workplace*. Available online at: http://theworkfoundation.com/DownloadPublication/Report/242_FINAL%20Why%20do%20employees%20come%20to%20work%20when%20ill.pdf (accessed 8.4.13).
13 http://www.dwp.gov.uk/health-work-and-well-being/case-studies (accessed 5.4.13).
14 WHO (2011) *Mental Health: A state of wellbeing*. Available online at: http://www.who.int/features/factfiles/mental_health/en/ (accessed 5.4.13).
15 Hefferon K, Boniwell I (2011) *Positive Psychology: Theory, research and applications*. Berkshire: Open University Press/McGraw–Hill Education.

16 Thornicroft G (2012) Global pattern of experienced and anticipated discrimination reported by people with major depressive disorder: A cross sectional study. *Lancet.* Available online at: http://press.thelancet.com/discrimination.pdf (accessed 5.4.13).

17 Thornicroft G (2006) *Actions Speak Louder Than Words: Tackling discrimination against people with mental illness.* Mental Health Foundation: Available online at: http://www.liv.ac.uk/media/livacuk/psssp/docs/actions_speak__louder1.pdf (accessed 5.4.13).

18 Sainsbury Centre for Mental Health (2009) 40: *Removing the Barriers: The facts about mental health and employment.* Available online at: http://www.centreformentalhealth.org.uk/pdfs/briefing40_Removing_barriers_employment_mental_health.pdf (accessed 5.4.13).

19 Karsay D (2011) *The Aspen Project: Anti stigma programme.* European Network. Work package 7.2: Barriers to Employment, Legal and social barriers to employment of people with psycho-social disabilities. Available online at: http://www.antistigma.eu/sites/default/files/ASPEN_WP7_BARRIERS_TO_EMPLOYMENT.pdf (accessed 5.4.13).

20 Kloss D, Ballard J (2012) *Discrimination Law and OH Practice.* London: The At Work Partnership.

21 www.timetochange.org.uk (accessed 23.11.12).

22 RobertsonCooper *Building Morale and Resilience: The key to surviving difficult times.* Available online at: www.robertsoncooper.com (accessed 12.4.13).

23 Clarke N, Macleod D (2009) *Engaging for Success: Enhancing performance through employee engagement.* Available online at: http://www.bis.gov.uk/files/file52215.pdf (accessed 5.4.13).

24 Robertson-Smith G, Markwick C (2009) *Employee Engagement: Summary.* A review of current thinking. Report 469. Institute for Employment Studies. Available online at: www.employment-studies.co.uk.

25 Business in the Community (2009) *Healthy People = Healthy Profits.* Available online at: www.bitc.org.uk (accessed 14.4.13).

26 TowersPerrin (2006) *Employee Wellbeing: Taking engagement and performance to the next level.* Available online at: www.bitc.org.uk (accessed 23.11.12).

27 Daniel Goleman (2004) *Emotional Intelligence: Working with emotional intelligence.* London: Bloomsbury.

28 Confederation of British Industry/Pfizer (2010) On the pathway to recovery; absence and workplace health survey 2010. London: CBI.

29 Towers Watson (2012) *Global Workforce Study. Engagement at risk: Driving strong performance in a volatile global environment.* Available online at: www.towerswatson.com.

30 Mowbray D (2013) *The Wellbeing and Performance Agenda.* Available online at: http://www.mas.org.uk/uploads/articles/Wellbeing_and_Performance_Agenda.pdf (accessed 5.4.13).

31 Mowbray D (2010) *The Manager's Code Connecting Wellbeing with Performance.* Available online at: www.mas.org.uk (accessed 14.3.13).

32 Health and Safety Executive/Chartered Institute of Personnel Development (2009) *Stress Management Competency Indicator Tool.* Available online at: www.hse.gov.uk (accessed 14.4.13).

33 The At Work Partnership (2005) Performance indicators and benchmarking in OH nursing. Available online at: www.atworkpartnership.co.uk (accessed 15.4.13).

34 http://www.hse.gov.uk/statistics/causdis/stress (accessed 5.4.13).

35 http://www.enwhp.org/toolbox/pdf/1007221128_Guidance%2520on%2520work-realted%2520stress.pdf (accessed 14.7.13).

36 http://www.hse.gov.uk/stress/index.htm (accessed 5.4.13).

37 http://www.isma.org.uk/about-stress/facts-about-stress (accessed 5.4.13).

38 Employment and social affairs (1999) *Health and Safety at Work: Guidance on work related stress – spice of life or kiss of death?* European Commission. Available online at: http://www.enwhp.org/toolbox/pdf/1007221128_Guidance%2520on%2520work-realted%2520stress.pdf (accessed 14.7.13).

39 Selye H (1956) *The Stress of Life.* New York: McGraw-Hill.

40 The Health and Social Care Information Centre (2009) *Adult Psychiatric Morbidity in England, 2007.* Results of a household survey. Available online at: https://catalogue.ic.nhs.uk/publications/mental-health/surveys/adul-psyc-morb-res-hou-sur-eng-2007/adul-psyc-morb-res-hou-sur-eng-2007-rep.pdf (accessed 16.4.13).

41 Lindsey J, Baillon S, Brugha T, Dennis M, Stewart R, Meltzer H (2006) Worry content across the lifespan: Analysis of 16–74 year old participants in the British National Survey of Psychiatric Morbidity, 2000. *Psychol Med* 36 (11): 1625–1633.

42 National Institute for Health and Clinical Excellence (2009) *Depression in Adults: The treatment and management of depression.* Available online at: http://www.nice.org.uk/nicemedia/pdf/CG90NICEguideline.pdf (accessed 5.4.13).

43 National Institute for Health and Clinical Excellence (2011) *Generalised Anxiety Disorder and Panic Disorder (with or without Agoraphobia) in Adults: Management in primary, secondary and community care.* Available online at: http://www.nice.org.uk/nicemedia/live/13314/52599/52599.pdf (accessed 5.4.13).

44 NICE (2011) *Common Mental Health Disorders: Identification and pathways to care.* CG123. Available online at: http://www.nice.org.uk/nicemedia/live/13476/54520/54520.pdf (accessed 5.4.13).

45 Royal College of Physicians (2010) *Depression Detection and Management of Staff on Long Term Sickness Absence: OH practice in the NHS in England: A national clinical audit round 2.* Available online at: http://www.rcplondon.ac.uk/sites/default/files/depression-detection-2010-national-audit-executive-summary_0.pdf (accessed 5.4.13).

46 Palmer K, Cox RAF, Brown I (2013) *Fitness for Work: The medical aspects,* 5th edn. Oxford: OUP.

47 Department of Health (2012) *Preventing Suicide in England: A Cross Government Outcomes Strategy to Save Lives.* London: Department of Health.

48 NICE (2009) *Promoting Mental Wellbeing at Work.* PH22. Available online at: http://www.nice.org.uk/nicemedia/live/12331/45893/45893.pdf (accessed 5.4.13).

49 Schneider J (2012) *Computerised CBT for Common Mental Health Disorders: RCT of a workplace intervention: Report to British Occupational Health Research Foundation.* Available online at: http://www.bohrf.org.uk/downloads/Computerised_CBT-Sep2012.pdf (accessed 5.4.13).

50 Guy K (2007) *Advance Statement for Service Users in a Mental Health Trust.* Available online at: www.nice.org.uk (accessed 16.4.13).

8 | Management of OH services

Andy Phillips

Learning objectives

After reading this chapter you will be able to:

- discuss the differences between organisational cultures within public- and private-sector companies
- appreciate the benefit of occupational health (OH) provision within public and private companies
- discuss what each stakeholder will require from their interaction with OH
- discuss the skills of communication needed for team working in a variety of business environments
- critically evaluate and understand resource management and collaborative working within organisations.

There have been many excellent chapters written by a variety of authors to describe the management of OH services. D'Auria,[1] one of the pioneers of OH education in Wales, described a statement from a well-known medical journal suggesting that OH was like Paris: it means different things to different people. Canvassing ideas from OH nursing students with regard to their thoughts on the content for this chapter suggested their views of management was similar to Paris.

This chapter aims to describe the different challenges that are faced by the OH practitioner in the delivery of OH services within a variety of different organisations. Types of organisation differ in size and sector and the chapter is written to reflect on some of the challenges that are faced by OH in differing businesses.

In order to decide on the level of support the company requires and to provide a bespoke OH service that attempts to integrate within the existing policies of the business, it is wise to undertake some form of OH needs assessment. This chapter will give guidance and examples of how to undertake such an assessment using a framework recommended by the National Institute for Health and Care Excellence (NICE).

Why do companies engage with OH services?

The Health and Safety Executive[2] has suggested that 'good health is good business' and there is growing evidence[3] which links employee wellbeing and health to business productivity. This has a major impact on the economic situation both organisationally and nationally. It should be acknowledged that, on the whole, there are a growing number of employers who are adopting measures aimed at promoting health and wellbeing amongst their employees.[4]

As Thornbory[5] rightly points out, employers want the maximum output for the minimum outlay. Yet, despite this main business principle, there are many who argue that this approach is simply not sustainable for businesses' longer-term survival. It has been shown that ignoring health-related issues can lead to not only serious economic consequences, but also increased sickness absence, threat of litigation and compensation costs, loss of reputation and increasing insurance premiums, all of which have huge ramifications on the business both financially and ethically. It is now thought by Bevan[6] that the approach to produce more for less can no longer be fully justified without looking at all of the variables relating to the health of the workforce which may impact on the business.

Black, in her report to the government on the health of the working-age population,[7] concluded that, amongst other things, UK employers are bearing the wider effects of ill health, chronic disease and health incapacity. Black argues that the situation is likely to get significantly worse over the next two to three decades as the workforce ages and as the incidence of chronic diseases increases; then employers will need to rethink their role in promoting wellbeing as both a business imperative and as part of their wider social responsibility.

D'Auria[1] suggests that, broadly, there are three strategic influences on the business's requirement for OH:

1. the legal requirements
2. professional advice
3. business issues.

Employers must remain compliant with the law. Companies, whatever the size, face a statutory duty to take reasonable care of the health of their employees. All employees who develop an illness related to their work can expect to hold their employer accountable. Employers' breaches of their statutory duties can lead to employees pursuing claims against their employers under either the criminal or civil justice systems. HSE can also enforce the law under the Health and Safety at Work Act 1974 by encouraging employers to bring about improvements to their health and safety practices. Failures to improve these health and safety practices can lead to health and safety improvement notices which, if not heeded, may lead to severe punishment by prosecution. Information regarding details of such prosecutions is available for others to see on the HSE website (http://www.hse.gov.uk/enforce/prosecutions.htm); these prosecutions carry large ramifications for the integrity and reputation of the business.[8]

Until recently, little was known about the extent to which employers choose to engage employee health services and the drivers behind the decision to initiate OH services. Miller and Haslam[9] conducted a qualitative study, in an attempt to understand the reasons why businesses engaged with OH services. As part of the study, they conducted interviews with 18 OH and safety professionals from a variety of industrial sectors from major organisations in the UK in order to understand the type of information that might be used to influence the business case for employee health. The study found that major businesses believe that promotion of employee health was seen as 'the right thing to do', as well as to assist the business to remain legally compliant.

Lian and Laing[10] suggest that there is an overall absence of sound cost benefit evaluation of the effects of the provision of OH services on the recipient business. In the absence of such information, they suggest that OH providers should focus on the promotion of employee health as an employee benefit as well as driving the message that the provision of OH services can improve the reputation of the company in receipt of the services.

Regardless of the reasons why companies engage OH services, it is suggested by the Chartered Institute of Personnel and Development (CIPD)[11] within their annual survey that, despite the current economic climate, companies remain committed to invest in the provision of workplace health and wellbeing. They suggest that nearly one-fifth of those surveyed had increased their wellbeing spend in the past year and nearly half of employers surveyed were continuing to invest the same amount of money in their wellbeing strategies. The survey also found that providing employees with access to counselling services (65 per cent) and assistance programmes (56 per cent) were the most common investments in workplace healthcare provision. More widely, the survey provided an indication of current absence trends. The average level of employee absence had fallen compared with 2011, from 7.7 to 6.8 days per employee per year. Yet this had coincided with almost one-third of employers reporting increased 'presenteeism', with more employees continuing to attend work despite feeling ill. The survey suggests that the increased threat of redundancy and concerns over job security were also contributing to this sharp rise in presenteeism. Stress-related absence continued to increase, with two-fifths of employers reporting a rise over the past year and just one in ten reporting a decrease, while stress remained the most common cause of long-term absence.

What size of company engages OH services?

In terms of structure, businesses come in a number of different shapes and sizes. To be clear from the outset, the Federation of Small Businesses (FSB)[12] defines small and medium enterprises (SMEs) as having less than 250 employees. Within this category, firms with less than 250 and more than 50 employees are regarded as medium-sized, 1–49 employees are small, whilst companies that employ fewer than ten people are defined as micro businesses. Larger businesses are those that employ more than 250 staff.

Micro, small and medium-sized enterprises currently represent a large majority of the overall economy. OH Advisory Committee[13] suggests that they employ 12.5 million people in the UK, which makes up approximately 99 per cent of all UK private-sector businesses, accounting for 54 per cent of industry turnover (excluding the finance sector) and 57 per cent of total employment. Small businesses are the source of just under half (45 per cent) of non-public-sector employment.

HSE[14] suggests that 82 per cent of all reported OH injuries occur within SMEs and, in some cases, these figures rise to 90 per cent of fatal accidents at work. Second, the CIPD draws a clear relationship between absence and the size of the workforce. FSB[15] suggests that SMEs are more likely to experience shorter-term absences due to minor ailments than their larger counterparts. Furthermore, there is evidence to suggest that smaller organisations are more likely to report lower absence levels than their larger counterparts, but this may be due to poor absence reporting rather than lower absences.

There are very few in-house OH services within SMEs as they may struggle to keep their heads above water regarding the best use of their income; one can also argue that there is no need to have such a fulltime professional OH service. Limited allocation of monies for external services such as health and safety, together with the high-risk nature of the work undertaken by some SMEs, particularly within the construction industry, means that there is still a gap in the provision of proactive health and safety risk prevention for employees. Despite evidence[16] that there is a general lack of management understanding within SMEs regarding the role of OH, managers within these types of business appear to be open to providing OH services to their employees. However, the costs of the services often influence the decision to engage with the OH services and, as such, any free or low-priced services are likely to be attractive to the sector.[17]

The delivery of OH services has received a certain degree of thought following studies from European models of service provision. Common themes across Europe include making OH provision mandatory, incentivising the use of OH through tax benefits for SMEs and reducing insurance premiums for small businesses. Black and Frost recommended such tax relief within their review of sickness absence in Britain.[18] In March 2013 the UK government announced in the budget that businesses will benefit from tax relief when they pay to help their employees return to the workplace after sickness. Within the new proposals, employers will receive tax relief on expenditure of up to £500 on health treatment recommended by a new health and work assessment and advisory service to support employees to return to work after a period of sick absence. Without this tax relief payments made on health-related interventions would be liable to income tax and employer National Insurance contributions. It is thought that this tax relief will encourage employers to fund around 110,000 health-related interventions to promote employee health.

Differences in business sector

Businesses broadly also fall within three sectors: public, private and voluntary. Public-sector companies are largely owned by either the government or its citizens, whether national or regional. Funded by taxation, these organisations are traditionally thought to meet commercial success criteria that are set out by the government, either centrally or locally.

Private-sector companies are those that are traditionally owned by private individuals or groups which often generate profit for financial gain in order to recoup investments, whether these be monetary, time or skills. Voluntary-sector companies, or the *not-for-profit sector*, are often not owned by the government, but fulfil unmet needs within society, and do not set out to make a profit.

To blur the lines somewhat, some small parts or whole services can be outsourced by public companies to private-sector firms, such as information technology or OH services. This means private organisations undertake work on behalf of, and funded by, the government.

Traditionally, there have been anecdotal tales within OH circles that there are stark differences in the way that OH is delivered by these types of organisation and how health and wellbeing are managed internally. In 2013 there was intense pressure from the UK government to make stringent efficiencies, downsizing or making cuts in all departments in an attempt to help remedy a global economic downturn; this rather predictably had a major effect on the public sector in that it needed to adapt to the situation. Departments and public bodies had to increase efficiency both within the organisations and with the employees working for them.[19] Boyne[20] highlighted the traditional view that public companies differ from their private counterparts because of differences in organisational environments, goals, structures and managerial values which require different management approaches. However, following an extensive review of 13 studies, it was found that there was insufficient evidence to support the notion that there were large differences between public- and private-sector companies. Interestingly, out of those differences there was significant evidence to support the anecdotal view that there are differences in human resources (HR) management policies and practices,[21] management of ethical issues and decision processes.

As a result, Mc Hugh[19] suggested that these efficiencies have driven changes within public-sector companies which include increased work targets, threat of job loss or redundancy, organisational change, changes in job holder's responsibilities and shifts in the balance of power between organisation and employee. These factors may lead to a potential rise in greater work-related pressures on employees which in turn was found in one study to affect employees' self-reported health adversely.[22]

In some ways, in terms of OH need, it is arguable that, in theory, all companies, regardless of size and sector, have similarities.

- They are all required to undertake the risk management process in order to protect the health of workers from work-related injury or illness.
- They are all likely to face similar consequences such as prosecution or improvement notices from the HSE, as mentioned above.
- They are all exposed to the potentially damaging effect on their business reputation if they fail to meet their legal obligations or to protect their employees' health.

As such, businesses of all sizes require the provision of similar services, whether they are SMEs or large multinational companies, e.g. they are all required to undertake risk assessments, monitoring of health, objective advice on employees with health problems and healthy living issues. The differences are with the practicalities of the actual day-to-day service provision and the way in which the services are delivered.

According to Bender and Joos-Vandewalle,[23] the most critical factor for the successful introduction of OH within any business is a firm and explicit public commitment by the employer's leaders that they have a caring philosophy. Thornbory,[5] however, realistically points out that in organisations, although there is a requirement for the employer to commit to these services, key purchasers of OH services are usually individuals, e.g. financial directors, HR, or health and safety managers within the organisation. If agreements exist between a single party within an organisation, for example, the HR department or health and safety managers, then often OH personnel are answerable to those persons directly, which OH professionals feel is often a threat to the independent role.

In all companies, it is important to undertake a *needs assessment* in order to decide on what type of OH support the business requires. Realistically, the company also has to decide on what provision it wants and how this can be achieved through its existing policies and procedures. Practically speaking, there can often be a dichotomy between what the company thinks are its priorities and what OH professionals believe the company needs are.

Health needs assessment

The Association of OH Nurse Practitioners UK argues that, in order to raise the profile of OH, and for companies to understand the importance of what we do, all OH nurses should promote themselves and their practice, their teams, their organisations and the profession when sharing good practice and engaging with stakeholders, customers and beneficiaries of the services. Put simply, as individuals, OH nurses need to believe in the value of what they are doing and integrate themselves in the businesses within the realms of their professional codes of conduct to enable mutual respect to be earned. 'We must seek to understand others before we can expect them to understand us.'[24]

An OH needs assessment provides the opportunity to gain such an awareness of the current health at work priorities of the workforce; to identify the gaps in healthcare provision; and to place recommendations to the organisation. The basis for the needs assessment will be set out below with a case study example at the end of the chapter. As stated above, many companies will wish to obey the law. When focusing on the legal requirements relating to the OH needs of the business, it is important for the practitioner to have an understanding of the principles of the Health and Safety at Work Act 1974[8] and those statutory regulations that are relevant to the work-related activities and risks which form part of the company profile. NICE defines health needs assessment as: 'A systematic method for reviewing the health issues facing a population, leading to agreed priorities and resource allocation that will improve health and reduce inequalities' (p. 3).[25]

There are many benefits to undertaking a health needs assessment:

- It provides the opportunity to identify the employees most at risk of work-related accidents or ill health in order to justify the reasons for choosing services, e.g. workers' exposure to vibration above the exposure action value and the need for assessment for hand–arm vibration syndrome (HAVS).

- It assists in the implementation of OH systems within an organisation or to review those already implemented.
- It enables the OH nurse to understand some of the social, economic and environmental influences on worker health within the company.
- It identifies any potential health problems which may affect the workforce and reviews what has already been done to overcome them.
- It encourages partnership working with many of the service users, such as line managers or employee representatives as part of the decision-making process.
- It helps to improve communication by gleaning information from those service users so that OH can justify the service or offer health interventions, e.g. health promotion activities (see Chapter 4).
- It promotes more efficient use of staff and resources within the OH department.

NICE[25] proposes a linear five-step approach to needs assessment (Figure 8.1), although it is recognised that some cross-checking may be required to ensure that each step is completed. All steps have been adapted to the OH setting using principles set out within *Health Needs Assessment: A practical guide.*[25] The process itself forms the basis of the assessment.

Step 1: Getting started

Before the OH needs assessment can be undertaken, it is fundamental that the company understands that it will need to provide the necessary information to glean any

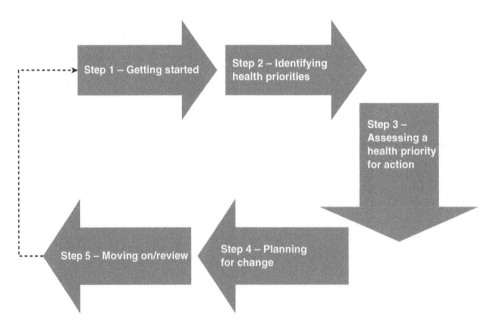

Figure 8.1 National Institute for Health and Clinical Excellence (NICE) five-step approach to needs assessment. Adapted from NICE (2005) *Health Needs Assessment: A practical guide.* London: NICE

gaps in health provision. To do this, one of the most critical components to successful assessment and provision of effective OH is a clear commitment and caring philosophy[25] from the company leadership, who 'buy in' to the process and recognise the need for the assessment so that the relevant information can become readily available to assist in the needs assessment process. As part of this, the company should have already fulfilled its legal obligation to undertake statutory risk assessments as part of the health and safety risk management process. This will enable the identification of any work-related threats and strategies would already be placed to overcome the adverse effect of the risk on the health of the worker from accidents or work-related ill health. This process is mentioned in Chapter 5.

When starting on the needs assessment, the population should be clearly identified and information given as to who should be contacted for the data required for the assessment. The population may involve the whole of the workforce, or a population of workers within the organisation, such as those within a particular department or a particular job type. It is possible that you may be able to gain the necessary information from the line managers, HR, health and safety, trade unions or the employees themselves. Once this has been established then the aims and objectives of the assessment should be clearly stipulated. Then, the resources and time required to undertake the health needs of the desired population should be considered. It is important to note that the assessment should be seen as worthwhile only if it benefits the organisation or those who work within it.[25]

Step 2: Identifying the health priorities

This step involves gathering the necessary data from the identified population. In terms of the OH needs assessment, this population profiling may contain information such as age, gender and numbers of migrant workers or those with disabilities. This health-related data may be gleaned from a variety of sources, including:

- HR, line management or electronically held data in order to obtain sickness absence statistics, including the absence trends (duration of absence) such as short- or long-term absence and the causes of these absences. Numbers of retirements due to ill health.
- Health and safety statistics: types and causes of work-related ill health or injuries, numbers of work-related ill health or injuries which result in lost time at work or those which necessitated reporting under the Reporting of Injuries, Diseases and Dangerous Occurrences Regulations (RIDDOR) 1995. Numbers of insurance claims for work-related ill health or injury.
- Epidemiology (see Chapter 9) and numbers of identified health conditions: obese workers, smokers, those with high blood pressure, stress or musculoskeletal conditions.
- Hold focus groups or workshops to find out the perceptions of health needs from those within the workplace, including workers, managers, trade unions, health and safety team, HR and not forgetting the current OH practitioners.
- Relevant national, regional, local health or organisational priorities.

Once the health profiling has been completed it will be necessary to prioritise the health issues according to the impact they have on the health of the workforce. For example, when collecting data there may be patterns emerging on the conditions which contribute to employee absence, work-related illness or accidents. The incidence of similar types of health problems from a variety of sources, such as musculoskeletal disorders, may highlight a problem in the workplace. For example, it may be noted that the incidence of musculoskeletal conditions is one of the main reasons for absence from work, as well as being one of the leading main reasons for insurance claims against the company. Furthermore, on interviewing, the OH nurse has referred many employees to the company physiotherapist with incidences of low-back problems; management notice that the employees are not using the assistive devices to enable them to undertake safe manual handling practices, but the employees claim that they have not received the training to do so. This may seem an extreme example, but hopefully it serves to illustrate the point. Once these health issues have been identified, it is important to identify the severity of the problem. One way that this can be done is to rank the health needs as having a high, medium and low severity for the organisation. This can then be evaluated and priorities of action established in the next step.

Step 3: Assessing a health priority for action

When determining how the health priorities can be addressed, it is important to focus on the main issues in the workplace that have the potential for the most impact on the organisation and the feasibility to bring about change, not forgetting that external factors may affect how feasible this is. When identifying the action priorities, consideration should be given to factors such as the size of the population that is affected, aspects which may have contributed to the action priority and whether there are any effective interventions.

For example:

- Some health priorities may be related to high-risk work, or may have statutory actions associated with them, such as medical surveillance associated with significant exposure to asbestos, or medicals for drivers of heavy goods vehicles.
- Some conditions may well have an established cause that impacts on the health of the worker, for example, exposure to noise greater than 85 dB leading to noise-induced hearing loss, or the effect of vibration exposure which may lead to HAVS.
- Consideration should be given to the underlying factors which contribute to the overall health and functioning of the workforce, for example, obesity or smoking.

Realistically, companies will say they want to obey the law but the feasibility of this with limited budgets or resources often means a 'belt and braces' approach to dealing with only those health issues which relate to the company's statutory obligations, or attending to those which have the potential to save the company money. Therefore there is sometimes a dichotomy between what the business thinks it needs and what the OH needs assessment actually recommends.

Step 4: Planning for change

This step involves setting clear, measurable aims and objectives on how to change the identified health priorities, and the action needed. This can be done by deciding on which health interventions may be the most appropriate. Sometimes, the OH practitioner may have evidence available to assist in this decision-making process. For example, when contemplating workplace health promotion strategies, there is evidence that is already available[26] to assist in the choice of effective health promotion strategies.

The stage involves making an action plan to assist in the delivery of the health intervention. It may be helpful at this stage to consider who the interventions are aimed at, how they will have a positive impact on the health outcome for the identified population and how the health outcome may be measured. The health intervention priorities should be clearly set out within the action plan. At this stage, the type of intervention should be clearly identified as well as the intended timescale for completion and identification of who will be responsible for the delivery and completion of the health intervention. For example, the identified health priority might be noise-induced hearing loss, which has been identified by the number of insurance claims the company has recently received, or even an improvement notice from HSE. The health intervention might require the implementation of a hearing conservation programme. Such a programme may involve audiometric testing by the OH nurse or OH technician in order to assess those who are showing signs of hearing loss. This will also provide anonymised trends to the health and safety team so that they can continue with preventing exposure to the noise using the principle of prevention (see Chapter 5).

Whilst planning the implementation of the health intervention, it is important to consider any potential barriers or problems that may be encountered at an early stage. This risk management strategy can help to minimise any delays in the health intervention. Once this has all been undertaken, the health intervention strategy should be implemented and monitored against the identified success criteria. For example, it would be prudent to monitor the impact of whether the audiometric screening programme has reduced the numbers of insurance claims or employee incidence of noise-induced hearing loss.

Step 5: Moving on/review

This part of the health needs assessment involves reflecting on the planning and delivery of the health intervention in order to evaluate and learn from the experience. When reflecting on the implementation of the health intervention, it is important to check the outcomes of the intervention against the initial aims and objectives in order to see whether the health intervention has been effective. Furthermore, there may be lessons learned from successes and failures which may affect the way that the health intervention is implemented next time.

Case study 8.1 Burns Boilers needs assessment – Siân Edwards

This report is the result of an OH needs assessment of Burns Boilers, which was conducted at the request of Burns Boilers to establish the type and level of OH service required. It is the result of a visit to the site which included a tour of the workshops, access to policies and procedures, sickness absence data, accident reports, insurance claims, Control of Substances Hazardous to Health (COSHH) data sheets and other information as requested. The visit also included discussion with the operations director, manufacturing manager, HR manager, safety manager, trade union representative and others.

The purpose of the report is to identify the OH needs of Burns Boilers and will inform any future negotiations of OH service provision between OH services and Burns Boilers.

Company background

Burns Boilers is an engineering company specialising in the manufacture, installation and servicing of industrial boilers. The main manufacturing site is in the Borders; there is an office in Leicester and field service engineers throughout the rest of the UK.

The Borders site has been established in a rural community for more than 80 years and they employ around 160 people. Of these, only 17 are female (all office-based). The majority of employees (around 130) are employed at the Borders site. The age range is from 19 to 66 with the majority of employees in the 45–60 age range. Approximately 50 employees are in support-type roles with over 100 employees directly involved in the manufacture, installation and servicing of boilers on site and in the field. A small number of staff work nights.

The manufacturing process includes cutting, shaping and extensive welding of metals. There is use of mineral wool insulation. There are elements of hot work; manual handling, including the use of cranes and other lifting aids; use of X-rays; confined-space work; vibration; noise; and working at height. The main hazard would appear to be from welding, particularly within confined spaces inside boilers.

Culture

There seems to be a culture of claims against the company. In the last year there have been six liability claims, mostly for HAVS, but also for accidents at work. In previous years there have also been claims for industrial deafness, mesothelioma and others. There is a culture of long hours with most people working overtime. A form for opting out of the maximum working-time 48-hour week (the Working Time

Regulations 1998) is sent out as standard to all new starters. Even office support workers routinely work 5–10 hours over their contracted hours each week. Personal protective equipment is taken seriously on site with both hearing protection and safety glasses mandatory on the workshop floor. However, it is unclear how that is enforced, as breaches have not routinely led to disciplinary action in the past.

Hazards to health

The site visit identified a number of hazards to health, many of which were already known to Burns Boilers. The main hazards identified were:

- weld fumes
- chemicals
- vibration
- confined-space work
- noise
- ionising radiation
- accidents (especially slips, trips and falls)
- manual handling
- work at height
- stress (including working long hours)
- lone working (including home visits and field work)
- driving at/for work (including outside working hours)
- overseas travel
- lead.

There is some asbestos on site but this is already registered and controlled.

There are a number of pieces of legislation which must be adhered to and health surveillance in this book is dealt with in depth in Chapter 5. However this case study specifically identifies the following to be relevant here: COSHH Regulations 2002; Control of Noise at Work Regulations 2005; Ionising Radiation Regulations 1999; Control of Lead at Work Regulations 2002. The health surveillance required includes skin, respiratory and audiometry surveillance; HAVS assessment; medical surveillance for work with lead, asbestos and ionising radiation.

Burns Boilers management were particularly concerned that HAVS screening and testing be carried out, ideally on site at Borders. There have been several previous liability claims and RIDDOR-reportable cases. A lot of work has been undertaken by Burns Boilers to assess and reduce the risk of HAVS. This includes changing tools and limiting trigger times.

There is evidence that working long hours over long periods of time can have a detrimental effect on health, including fatigue, psychological effects and general

(continued)

(continued)

health.[27] Driving and operating machinery whilst fatigued can increase the risk of accidents. This should be taken into account whilst planning workloads and overtime. Fatigue from long hours can contribute to sickness absence rates.

OH needs

Apart from health surveillance, there were other OH needs identified during the assessment, including:

- maintaining OH records; reporting to management and statutory health records for COSHH, lead and Ionising Radiation Regulations
- pre-employment/preplacement screening
- fitness to work (includes night work; fork lift truck driving; work at height; confined space; display screen equipment use; retirement/older workers)
- occupational travel health advice
- sickness absence (including advice on Equality Act, rehabilitation, referral to specialist services and adjustments)
- health and safety meetings (management and trade union were both keen for OH to be involved)
- assisting in risk assessments (including manual handling, stress, pregnancy)
- policies and procedures
- drug and alcohol
- training (including first aid; manual handling; stress)
- health promotion.

The Nursing and Midwifery Council and Faculty of Occupational Medicine have guidelines for record keeping and confidential OH records will be maintained in accordance with those guidelines (see Chapters 5 and 6). OH services would also be able to keep a database for health surveillance, offering automatic recalls and ensuring that statutory requirements for health surveillance are met. They will also be able to carry out clinical audit to ensure quality and excellence.

On-employment screening is currently carried out by paper-screening health questionnaires. Any positive responses on the questionnaire are then followed up. It may be necessary to undertake a medical for new starters in the future to obtain a baseline for future health surveillance. This could incorporate drug and alcohol testing in line with properly approved local policy if they are adopted. Although the bulk of on-employment screening is likely to be carried out at the Borders site, OH services have the capability to undertake this around the country if necessary (e.g. for field service engineers).

There is no current provision for health checks for night workers. The Working Time Regulations 1998 say that night workers are entitled to a health check prior to starting night work and at regular intervals (usually annually). If night workers do not have any other health check through health surveillance programmes then a questionnaire may be administered to fulfil this requirement with follow-up for any positive responses.

HSE guidance on fitness to drive recommends that workers involved in workplace transport (including fork lift trucks) should be screened at pre-employment. Once they reach the age of 40 the guidance recommends regular fitness assessments every 5 years. Currently there is no formal assessment of fitness to drive, although this can be incorporated into the annual health surveillance medical.

The Health and Safety (Display Screen Equipment) Regulations 1992 give users and occasional users the right to regular eye and eyesight checks. OH can provide a screening service to help minimise the cost of specialist eye examinations. They can also assist in workstation assessments and advise on ergonomics in the workplace, including recommendations for specialist equipment where required.

There is currently no requirement for assessment of fitness for working at height or in confined spaces. There is work under way by Burns Boilers to address the risks of working at height and assessment of fitness for such work would be a logical step. Assessing fitness for confined-space work would also be logical. It may also be necessary to review the risk assessment for confined-space work, particularly with regard to supervision of workers undertaking confined-space work and emergency procedures. The assessment of fitness for work at height and/or in confined spaces would include musculoskeletal assessment as well as general health, including cardiovascular, neurological, mental health and metabolic conditions.

One of the key roles of OH, and one with considerable cost benefit, is in sickness absence management. Estimates of cost benefit range from 1:3 to 1:12[7] with savings of £3–12 for every £1 spent on sickness absence management services. Linked to this service would be assistance in developing the sickness absence management policy; training for managers on how to manage sickness absence and how and when to refer; assessing individuals and advising on fitness, return to work programmes and possible adjustments; referral to specialists if necessary; and advice on disability, ill-health retirement and capability as appropriate.

OH can provide travel health advice for employees required to undertake occupational travel overseas. This includes advice on flying, vaccinations, malaria prophylaxis, safe sex, food and drink, sun protection and first aid.

There is currently only a draft policy for retirement. The retirement age has been set at the default 65 years and only in special circumstances can employees apply to continue working past retirement. There is currently no requirement for an assessment of fitness to continue work. Nor is there provision of health checks for older workers (Arnold (2008)[28] cites World Health Organization

(continued)

(continued)

recommendations that all workers over 45 should be offered annual health assessments). Approximately 58 per cent of the workforce of Burns Boilers falls into this group. Annual health surveillance would suffice for those who require it. For those workers not under health surveillance programmes, annual health questionnaires may be administered, with follow-up for positive responses.

OH can assist in the development of policies and procedures related to health, safety and wellbeing. Several policies are in draft form at present but have yet to be adopted by Burns Boilers. OH can assist in the development of these policies, including stress; sickness absence; hearing conservation; and substance abuse.

There are a number of external agencies able to offer support with training and updates for first aid. 'The Health and Safety (First-Aid) Regulations 1981 require employers to provide adequate and appropriate equipment, facilities and personnel to enable first aid to be given to employees if they are injured or become ill at work.'[29] OH services can advise on selection of appropriate providers if required.

Other training, which could be provided by OH services, might include:

- manual handling training (including for support staff)
- sickness absence management training for managers
- stress management awareness and specific training for managers on stress risk assessment
- drug and alcohol awareness training and training in drug and alcohol testing if required
- training of responsible person for skin surveillance
- toolbox talks could be tailored in line with local workplace hazards.

Burns Boilers management were reluctant to divert resources from the statutory requirements towards voluntary health promotion activities. However, there is a clear role for OH in promoting health. This includes *ad hoc* advice, poster campaigns and formal events. Health promotion can benefit the business by helping to improve the general health and wellbeing of the workforce. An early health promotion event would also serve to raise the profile of the OH service which can improve the uptake and effectiveness of the service. OH services will take every opportunity afforded to it to promote health.

Resources

The current suggested level is 21 OH visits per year.

Approximately 80–90 employees at the Borders site will require health surveillance of some type. This alone equates to 12 nurse clinics per year. Further nurse time will be required for sickness absence cases, and some physician time will also be required for complex sickness absence cases as well as statutory medicals for COSHH, radiation and lead. Further clinical time will be required for satellite services, providing health surveillance and sickness absence management to field engineers and other remote workers. Some nurse time will also be needed for attending health and safety meetings and other non-clinical aspects of the service. Specialist nurse practitioner time will be required to deal with strategic needs such as assisting in the development of policies and procedures and contract management. It is suggested that a review is held once a month for the first 3 months to evaluate the service and to tailor the service as necessary. If all is well then quarterly contract reviews may suffice.

It is suggested then that the service include:

- 18–24 nurse days per year (not necessarily all at Borders)
- six specialist nurse practitioner days per year
- six physician days per year
- *ad hoc* provision of training.

Burns Boilers has now provided a treatment room in the main admin area which is suitable for OH use. The room has frosted windows and blinds; a desk; filing cabinets; and a small sink. Further equipment such as a couch and screen and scales may also be beneficial. Alternative arrangements should be made for first-aid treatment during the times when the treatment room is in use by the OH service. Consideration should be given to the provision of more specialised equipment such as audiometer, spirometer and vision screener, although OH services can provide equipment for use during their clinics. Access to suitable toilet facilities may be required if drug and alcohol testing is introduced, depending on the type of testing. Consideration should also be given to the provision of consumables such as record forms, disposable mouthpieces, examination gloves and urinalysis sticks.

Case study conclusion and recommendations

The main OH needs of Burns Boilers are:

- health surveillance
- sickness absence management
- fitness-for-work assessments, including pre-employment, and reports to management
- maintenance of confidential OH records and provision of statutory health surveillance records
- strategic development of policies and procedures
- training
- health promotion.

Delivery of OH services

D'Auria[1] suggests that there is no generally accepted definition of what constitutes an OH service and no clear single form of practice, but such services are traditionally understood to be medically based and led by doctors or nurses. The Faculty of Occupational Medicine[30] has suggested that SMEs do not necessarily require a traditional doctor-and-nurse-based service but could benefit from simple, sector-specific guidance on practical measures, with the aim being to improve health and to prevent health risks at work and those issues that surround the effects of health at work. As a result of this, alternative frameworks have been recommended, to include the establishment and provision of OH helplines and websites for those requiring OH support, including an NHS Plus SME helpline, the Constructing Better Health scheme, Scotland's health at work SME toolkit and both the Welsh and English SME helplines.

Whatever the mode of delivery, the provision of OH services can make a large difference to the health and productivity of the employees within the business.

According to Fingret and Smith,[31] OH services traditionally include:

- the assessment of fitness to work, including rehabilitation, advice on resettlement or retirement on the grounds of ill health
- assistance in the implementation of health and safety legislation: assisting in risk assessments, ergonomic assessments, undertaking statutory examinations, medical surveillance or screening, accident review
- health promotion: development of policies, workshops, literature or campaigns
- stress management: provision of counselling or workplace support
- arrangements for early treatment interventions such as physiotherapy.

When organisations wish to engage OH services they can choose whether this is offered 'in-house', where the service is delivered by their own staff, or delivered via an external provider. Bray[32] highlighted the criteria that can sometimes be used to select external OH providers, including:

- geographical coverage
- cultural fit
- areas of expertise
- proactivity spectrum of services
- knowledge of the market
- ability to manage contractual relationships
- cost.

According to Bray,[32] employer complaints about OH services delivered by providers include:

- They don't understand our business.
- Advice is not commercial and is often indecisive, with providers tending to sit on the fence.

- We have to chase the provider for reports and outcomes following consultations.
- They deliver the service to suit themselves, with poor levels of communication.
- Return-to-work plans are not discussed with HR.
- The management information is poor.
- The services, such as employee assistance programmes and OH, are working in isolation.
- The service is patchy across the country.
- In-house OH services require a lot of internal management.

According to Everton,[33] the business case for the procurement of OH services will include a specification to describe the needs of the service, the desired cost and how the service is to be delivered. Once the provider has been chosen, it is necessary that a Service Level Agreement (SLA) contract is drafted that clearly states and regulates what is expected between both parties, and what legal recourse there is if this contract is not satisfied. A template example of an SLA contract relating to OH services was launched by NHS Health at Work and is available for download at: http://www.nhsemployers. org/SiteCollectionDocuments/Template_NHS_SLA_final_22062012.doc.

Key Performance Indicators (KPIs) is a term which is used to define and measure performance towards organisational goals. An organisation may use KPIs to evaluate the success of the organisation as a whole, or a particular activity in which the client engages. KPIs need to be measurable and focus on a range of areas within the service provision.

Examples of KPIs include:

- the time between referral and the provision of the OH advisory report
- numbers of employees attending appointments
- customer satisfaction
- service quality.

Standards of service have developed into a rather hot topic of late: one of the largest influences to affect standards in the delivery of OH services in recent years was recommended by Black.[7] Black suggested that OH providers should adhere to clear standards of practice, a factor that was endorsed by the government in its response,[34] published shortly after the report. To take this concept forward, a stakeholder group that was led by the Faculty of Occupational Medicine was set up to develop Standards of Accreditation for OH services.[35] These standards were launched as SEQOHS (Safe Effective Quality Occupational Health Service) in January 2010 and provide six domains for OH providers to achieve:

1. business probity (standards with regard to the integrity of the business and the propriety of its financial affairs)
2. information governance (standards in relation to the adequacy of records and maintenance of confidentiality)
3. people (standards in relation to the competency and supervision of OH staff)
4. facilities and equipment (ensuring that facilities are safe, accessible and appropriate to the client group which OH serves)

5. relationships with purchasers (the ability of the provider to provide a fair service with a customer focus)
6. relationships with workers (fair treatment, respect and involvement of the workers within the business).

Conclusion

There are many factors that need to be taken into account when managing OH services and the way in which OH services are going to be managed will continue to change as time goes on. Recent innovations in service delivery may challenge the way in which OH will be delivered to organisations in the future.

OH service delivery has the potential to undergo radical change following proposals set out within the Black and Frost report[18] and was endorsed by the government's response to the review.[36] The government's intention to establish a Health and Work Assessment and Advisory service in 2014 is generally seen as a positive step for OH. However, before a new service is commenced there have been calls to clarify how this service can be managed and what the strategy will actually look like. Despite this, it is hoped that by gaining an understanding of the differences of OH provision for a variety of organisations, OH nurses will be VIPs, as Butterworth et al.[24] suggest: visible, informed and positive.

References

1 D'Auria D (2002) OH systems. In: Hawkins L (ed.) *Guide to Managing Employee Health*. Croydon: Lexis Nexis.
2 Health and Safety Executive (1999) *Good Health is Good Business*. HSE Books. Available online at: http://www.occ-med.co.uk/ghgb4.pdf (accessed 25.03.13).
3 Hill D, Lucy D, Tyers C, James L (2007) *What Works at Work? Review of the evidence assessing the effectiveness of workplace interventions to prevent and manage common health problems. Corporate Document Services*. Available online at: http://www.employment-studies.co.uk/pdflibrary/whwe1107.pdf (accessed 25.03.13).
4 Business in the Community (BITC) 2009 *Healthy People = Healthy Profits*. Available online at: http://www.bitc.org.uk/our-resources/report/healthy-people-healthy-profits (accessed 25.03.13).
5 Thornbory G (2009) *Public Health Nursing: A textbook for health visitors, school nurses and OH nurses*. London: Wiley-Blackwell.
6 Bevan S (2010) *The Business Case for Employees' Health and Wellbeing: A report prepared for Investors in People*. London: The Work Foundation.
7 Black C (2008) *Working for a Healthier Tomorrow*. London: TSO. Available online at: http://www.dwp.gov.uk/docs/hwwb-working-for-a-healthier-tomorrow.pdf.
8 Hawkins L (2002) *Guide to Employee Health*. Croydon: Lexis Nexis.
9 Miller P, Haslam C (2009) Why employers spend money on employee health: Interviews with OH and safety professionals from British industry. *Saf Sci* 47: 163–169.
10 Lian PCS, Laing AW (2007) Perception and provision of OH services in the UK. *Occup Med* 57: 472–479.

11 Chartered Institute of Personnel and Development (CIPD) (2012) *Absence Management Survey.* Available online at http://www.cipd.co.uk/research/_absence-management (accessed 19.04.13).

12 Federation of Small Businesses (2008) *Small Businesses in the UK: New perspectives on evidence and policy.* Available online at: http://www.fsb.org.uk/policy/images/fsbwestminster01%2012%20(3).pdf (accessed 19.04.13).

13 OH Advisory Committee (2009) *Report and Recommendations on Improving Access to Occupational Health Support.* Available online at: http://www.hse.gov.uk/aboutus/meetings/iacs/ohac/access.htm (accessed 20.03.13).

14 HSE (2006) RR504 – Six SME case studies that demonstrate the business benefit of effective management of occupational health and safety. Norwich: HMSO. Available online at: http://www.hse.gov.uk/research/rrpdf/rr504.pdf.

15 Federation of Small Businesses (2006) Health matters: The small business perspective. London: Federation of Small Businesses. Available online at: http://www.fsb.org.uk/policy/images/fsb%20health%20matters%20report.pdf.

16 HSE (2004). Report RR257. Occupational Health and SMEs: focused intervention strategies. Norwich: HMSO. Available online at: http://www.hse.gov.uk/research/rrpdf/rr257.pdf.

17 Phillips A (2011) *Why Should SMEs Invest in OH?* Available online at: http://www.personneltoday.com/articles/01/07/2011/57551/why-should-smes-invest-in-occupational-health.htm (accessed 13 March 2013).

18 Black C, Frost D (2011) *Health at Work – Independent review of sickness absence.* HMSO. Available online at: https://www.gov.uk/government/uploads/system/uploads/attachment_data/file/181060/health-at-work.pdf (accessed 20.03.13).

19 McHugh M (1998) Rationalisation is a key stressor for public sector employees: An organisational case study. *Occup Med (Lond)* 48 (2): 103–112.

20 Boyne GA (2002) Public and private management: What's the difference? *J Manage Studies* 39 (1): 97–122.

21 Boyne GA, Jenkins G, Poole M (1999) Human resource management in the public and private sectors: An empirical comparison. *Public Administration* 77: 407–420.

22 Iwi D, Watson P, Barber N, Kimber N, Sharman G (1998) The self-reported well-being of employees facing organisational change: Effects of an intervention. *Occup Med* 48 (6): 361–368.

23 Bender and Joos-Vandewalle (2013) Corporate and in-house OH services. Cited in: Gudotti TL, Arnold S, Luksco DG, Green McKenzie J, Bender J, Rothstein MA, Leone FH, OHara K, Stecklow M *OH Services: A practical approach*, 2nd edn. London: Routledge.

24 Butterworth C, Henderson J, Minshell C (2008) Be a VIP. *Occup Hlth* 60 (8): 32–33.

25 National Institute for Health and Clinical Excellence (NICE) (2005) *Health Needs Assessment: A practical guide.* Available online at: http://www.nice.org.uk/media/150/35/Health_Needs_Assessment_A_Practical_Guide.pdf.

26 Meyrick J (ed.) (1998) *Effectiveness of Health Promotion Interventions in the Workplace: A review.* Available online at http://www.nice.org.uk/nicemedia/documents/effective_workplace.pdf.

27 White J, Beswick J (2003) *Working Long Hours.* Sheffield: Health and Safety Laboratory. Available online at: http://www.hse.gov.uk/research/hsl_pdf/2003/hsl03-02.pdf.

28 Arnold, H (2008) Occupational health and the ageing workforce. *Occup Hlth.* Available online at: http://www.personneltoday.com/articles/08/04/2008/44171/occupational-health-and-the-ageing-workforce.htm#.UeBmIMr-vh4.

29 HSE (2009) *The Health and Safety (First-Aid) Regulations 1981: Approved code of practice and guidance.* Norwich: TSO. Available online at: http://www.hse.gov.uk/pubns/priced/l74.pdf.

30 Faculty of Occupational Medicine (2006) *Position Statement: Provision of occupational health services to small and medium enterprises.* London: Faculty of Occupational Medicine.
31 Fingret A, Smith A (1995) *OH: A practical guide for managers.* London: Routledge.
32 Bray C (2008) Safety nets. *Occup Hlth* 60 (5): 26–27.
33 Everton S (2012) Contracts for OH services. *Occup Hlth* 64 (11): 26–30.
34 UK government (2008) *Improving Health and Work: Changing lives.* The government`s response to Dame Carol Black's review of the Health of Britain's Working Age Population. Available online at: http://www.dwp.gov.uk/docs/hwwb-improving-health-and-work-changing-lives.pdf (accessed 30.04.13).
35 Faculty of Occupational Medicine (2010) *OH Service Standards for Accreditation*, *London.* Available online at: https://www.seqohs.org/DocumentStore/fom_seqohs.pdf (accessed 30.04.13).
36 Department for Work and Pensions (2013) *Fitness for Work: The government response to 'Health at Work – an independent review of sickness absence'.* Available online at: https://www.gov.uk/government/uploads/system/uploads/attachment_data/file/181072/health-at-work-gov-response.pdf (accessed 28.04.13).

9 Epidemiology and research

Diane Romano-Woodward

Learning objectives

After reading this chapter you will be able to:

- explain what is meant by epidemiology
- appreciate the importance of research to practice in occupational health (OH)
- describe types of research
- discuss and appreciate research in order to incorporate it into OH practice.

This chapter aims to provide a basic introduction to the principles, methods and applications of epidemiology and research in public health and specifically in OH. It aims to prepare OH nurses for an approach to healthcare that is increasingly concerned with preventive medicine and the most efficient use of resources. It will show how the tools of epidemiology can be applied to the prevention of disease, the promotion of health and the formulation of policies. Particular attention is given to the use of epidemiological research to detect associations between modifiable environmental factors and specific diseases. In order to do this it is important to understand what is meant by epidemiology and research as well as its importance in OH practice.

Epidemiology

This is derived from the Greek *epi*, 'upon', *demos*, 'people' and *logos*, 'study'. It is widely accepted now that environmental factors, such as physical and chemical exposures, and also biological, sociological and political processes can have an effect upon the health of individual; this has been demonstrated in Chapters 2, 4, 5 and 7 covering public health, health promotion, health surveillance and mental health.

Hippocrates observed over 2,000 years ago that such factors influence the occurrence of disease.[1] Centuries later, Ramazzini identified some of these factors in relation to the health problems associated with the occupations of workers.[2] Epidemiology is concerned with disease, or any unfavourable health change, including injury and mental wellbeing, disability and death. It also examines positive health states and the ways to bring them about.[1] A formal definition of epidemiology is 'the study of the distribution of determinants of health-related states or events in specified populations and the application of this study to the prevention and control of health problems'.[1]

Research

Research is an activity undertaken to develop and to contribute to knowledge in order to improve practice. The intended beneficiaries of the research will include those under study, but will always extend beyond them to society and the data collected exceed the requirement for care. The information is gathered in a systematic way to reduce bias, allowing it to be relevant beyond the programme from which it was collected; that is, different settings and populations.[3]

Practising with evidence

However, simply because relevant research and evidence-based guidance exist, this does not mean that they will be used to improve practice. The Health Development Agency has indicated some of the barriers in getting evidence into public health[4] (Figure 9.1).

The UK government has developed strategies to tackle public inequalities in health. The NHS Plan in 2000 identifies a number of key elements that would contribute to reducing health inequalities,[5] including an evidence-based approach. The Health Development Agency (now part of the National Institute for Health and Care Excellence (NICE)) was set up to assist the efforts in tackling health inequalities, so that organisations and individual practitioners would be able to base their work on the highest standards. It was felt that this would have the long-term effect of raising the quality of the public health function in England. The approach was along the lines of evidence-based clinical medicine. This has been defined as the 'the conscious, explicit and judicious use of current best evidence in taking decisions about the individual patients'.[6] Using evidence from primary research, explicit guidance was produced through systematic reviews or secondary research. Primary research is based on randomised controlled trials, and this is appropriate to determine the effectiveness of drug interactions and treatments. This may not be an appropriate research method for evaluating complex community-based interventions where target groups cannot be randomised to produce controls. Indeed, in the community there are simultaneous multiple interventions operating on individuals and communities and at system levels. In these situations randomised controlled trials might be 'unnecessary, inappropriate, impossible or inadequate to provide evidence of effectiveness'.[7] This will be explored later in the chapter. Even with reliable evidence and guidance, bringing about change based on evidence is unreliable. Knowledge transfer does not happen according to simple cause and effect, and making information available to practitioners does not necessarily or automatically lead to its adoption and a change in practice. Schaafsma

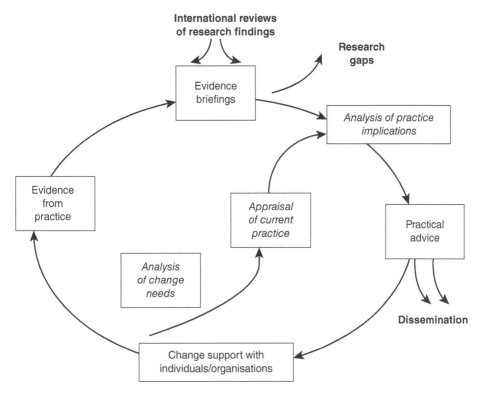

Figure 9.1 Getting evidence into practice in public health

Source: Health Development Agency (2004) *Getting Evidence into Practice in Public Health*. Available from www.nice.org.uk. Reproduced with permission.

et al.[8] reviewed the extent and nature of information demands of 159 OH physicians in the Netherlands. In their questions concerned with medical, legal and rehabilitation topics in particular they found that to obtain answers they generally chose to contact colleagues. They found that scientific databases were not consulted often, although, in general, the attitude towards evidence-based medicine was positive.

For evidence to be directly applied in the field, an active approach to making it accessible, placed in context and usable is required before it will be implemented. This can be in the form of action briefings, new tools, resources and educational material, including the use of electronic networks.[9] For example, the British Occupational Health Foundation published evidence-based guidance on occupational asthma in 2005.[10] Members of the working party produced the main guidance plus three leaflets, aimed at employers/employees, general practitioners (GPs)/practice nurses and OH professionals. There were articles produced for the appropriate journals for practitioners of OH and medicine, safety, respiratory medicine, GPs and practice nurse, as well as free online training for GPs. There were also study days to launch the guidance and it was publicised at conferences.

That nurses practising in OH should be using research and evidence to justify their practices is entrenched in the *Standards of Proficiency for Specialist Community Public Health Nurses*:

Within the complex and rapidly changing environment for specialist community public health nurses, it is essential that practice is informed by the best available evidence. This commitment is reflected in the standards of proficiency. It includes searching the evidence base, analysing, critiquing, using research and other forms of evidence in practice, and disseminating research findings and adapting practice where necessary. The ability to synthesise new knowledge into practice, applying it to all areas of work where it is relevant and likely to be effective, must be reflected throughout all programmes of preparation.[11]

Additionally many OH services aspire to demonstrating that they provide a service of a specific quality. When being assessed against the standards for Safe, Effective, Quality Occupational Health Services (SEQOHS), there is a requirement for all OH services (other than single-handed practitioners) to: 'demonstrate clinical governance and maintain documented protocols that ensure the delivery of services that reflect current evidence based guidelines, national guidelines and Approved Codes of Practice.'[12]

Evidence may also be useful in observing trends in occupational disease and suggesting what might be appropriate to include in the training of OH nurses and doctors. Alessio et al.[13] review the notes of 9,080 individuals referred to a specialist centre in occupational medicine in Brescia, Italy. Of these, 3,759 were found to have occupational diseases: allergic skin disease (23.4 per cent), pneumoconiosis (20.4 per cent), chronic obstructive pulmonary disease (15.9 per cent), noise hearing loss (7.1 per cent), musculoskeletal disorders (6.9 per cent), respiratory allergies (6.9 per cent), cancer (5.9 per cent) and miscellaneous (6.4 per cent). When consideration was given to the previous 5-year period, there was a definite increase in musculoskeletal disorders, cancer and, to a lesser extent, diseases due to psychosocial factors. The authors concluded that the frequency of traditional occupational diseases is progressively lowering, their gravity is decreasing and the etiological factors are changing. This was felt to be relevant in influencing what is included in the curriculum for OH professionals, but also to indicate the most relevant topics to be addressed with future research.

Sources of evidence-based guidance

Practitioners in OH will be aware of sources of evidence-based guidance such as the NICE,[14] British Occupational Health Research Foundation[15] and the Health and Safety Executive (HSE).[16] The NHS has set up an online clinical benchmarking tool that is designed to help OH teams in the NHS raise standards of health service at work. This is called MoHaWK (short for Management of Health at Work Knowledge) and it has created evidence-based guidelines on seven topics relevant to workers in the NHS.[17] In addition several colleges of medicine have produced guidance on medical procedures, recovery and returning to work which are relevant to OH practice. This includes the Royal College of Physicians' (RCP) health and work development unit, which is a partnership between the RCP and the Faculty of Occupational Medicine.[18] Other sources of guidance can be found in the Appendix.

Finding research relevant to a health issue

There will be occasions when no evidence-based guidance has been produced, and the practitioner will need to source and interpret research and decide on its applicability. In order to find out what has already been discovered about the topic of interest a search is undertaken of relevant databases. An overview of this process can be found on the Royal College of Nursing website,[19] where there is information and also the provision of webinars to give an overview of the topic. Suitable databases include the British Nursing Index, Cumulative Index to Nursing and Allied Health Literature (CINAHL), ProQuest Nursing and Allied Health Source, Medline, the Allied and Complementary Medicine Database (AMED), the Health Management Information Consortium (HMIC), the Department of Health (DH-Data) and The Cochrane Database.[20,21] Guidance on how to undertake a systematic review in OH has been provided by Nicholson[22] and a search strategy for OH intervention studies in Medline has been produced by Verbeek *et al.*[23]

An indepth explanation of statistics falls outside the scope of this chapter but there are several online resources which will assist. In particular, the *British Medical Journal* has compiled a collection of useful online resources,[24] some of which give an understanding of basic statistics and types of research.[25,26] These can also be found in nursing journals,[27,28] books[29] and online training.[30] However it is useful to understand the basics.

Statistics

When we are looking at information about groups, we note it in the form of observations. If there is a numerical value attached to the observation or it is measured in some way, it is called a quantitative observation. Examples of this are height, weight, body mass index, blood lead levels, forced vital capacity in spirometry and hearing threshold limit in decibels in audiometry. If the measurement is based on an act of recognition, and allocating different diagnoses to a category, e.g. male or female, then the observations are called qualitative.[31]

When observations are made in large numbers it is useful to be able to describe the whole set rather than each individual observation. Concepts such as averages, percentages, graphs and figures may be useful.

Quantitative data

A set of measurements can be shown as a distribution, in the form of a table or a figure. Along the horizontal axis the value of the measurement is represented. Along the vertical axis is the number of observations in that class. This is called a histogram. At times it is more useful to group the individual measurements into classes. The grouping of the data can happen as it is collected, for example weight rounded up to the nearest kilogram and recorded, or it can be done at a later stage, so weight is recorded to a set number of decimal places and then grouped later.

A frequency distribution is comprehensive but may not be a convenient way of describing a population. It may be appropriate to make a summary of certain characteristics such as a central value, or by an indication of the shape of the distribution. These are known as summarising statistics or parameters of the distribution.

Indicators of the central tendency are the mean, median and mode. The mean is calculated by adding up all the values of the observations and dividing it by the number of observations. The median is the value of the observation which has half of the observations below it and half above. The mode is the value which occurs most frequently, and in a histogram it is the tallest column. In a symmetrical distribution, the mean, median and mode are the same value. Many biological parameters such as blood pressure and height follow this pattern, which resembles a theoretical mathematical curve known as normal or Gaussian distribution. This symmetrical curve is bell-shaped, convex at the top and concave at both ends (Figure 9.2).

Understanding the spread of the distribution can be useful. The range of the situation is the interval between the highest and lowest value. For example, in a normal person, the range of the blood sugar level before a meal is 4.0–5.9 mmol/l.[32] However this is not of great value as it is usually only two readings and these may be the most extreme and least reliable.

It may be more useful to know the percentiles of the distribution. This is the value below which a certain percentage of the values lie. The median is the 50th percentile, and the 25th percentile is also known as a quartile, as a quarter of the values lie below it. The 75th percentile is the quartile above which 25 per cent of the values lie. Other useful values are the 5th percentile and the 95th percentile.

The standard deviation (SD) is a useful index of the spread of a symmetrical distribution as each individual observation contributes to it. When looking at a value, one can consider how far this value is from the central value or mean. The distance from any value to the mean is called the deviation, and this can be positive or negative depending on whether the value is greater than or less than the mean. As simply adding these numbers would lead to the cancelling effect of the positive and negative numbers, the values are squared to produce all positive numbers. These are then added up and the mean is found, to produce the mean square deviation. Taking the square root

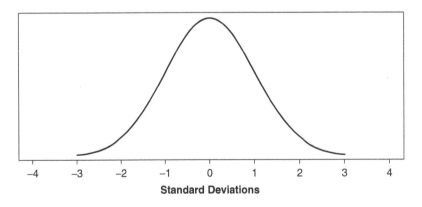

Standard Deviations

Figure 9.2 Standard deviations

of the mean square deviation produces the standard deviation. When looking at a normal distribution, about two-thirds of the values can be found to lie within 1 SD above and below the mean and 95 per cent of the values can be found to lie within approximately 2 SD of the mean. (The actual value is ±1.96 SD of the mean.[33] This will become relevant when considering probability.) If the SD is small then the distribution of the values is likely to be tightly packed around the mean, with large differences occurring infrequently. If the SD is large, large differences from the mean are likely to be found.

Types of studies

There are a variety of ways to look at health issues and the factors affecting them.[34] In epidemiology, studies investigate the distribution and historical changes in the frequency of diseases and what might cause these changes. They include both interventional (or experimental) studies and non-interventional (or observational) studies.

Interventional studies are further subdivided into field studies (sample from an area, such as a large region or a country) and group studies (sample from a specific group, such as a specific social or ethnic group).

Randomised controlled trials

These are occasionally found in the OH setting. They answer questions about the effectiveness of different care options, or control measures.

Example of a randomised controlled trial
Williams *et al.*[35] described a study where 132 healthy adult volunteers who worked in healthcare were randomly allocated to use one of five different moisturising lotions or soap alone when washing hands approximately 15 times a day. This was a 'double-blind' trial, meaning that neither the subjects of the experiment nor the persons administering the experiment know the critical aspects of the experiment, in this case which moisturising lotion was being supplied. A double-blind procedure is used to guard against both experimenter bias and placebo effects. The effect on skin barrier function was determined by assessment after repeated hand washing over a 2-week period. Assessments of transepidermal water loss, epidermal hydration and a visual assessment using the Hand Eczema Severity Index were made at days 0, 7 and 14. The authors found that there was a significant worsening of the clinical condition of the skin in those who washed their hands without using moisturiser, whereas there was no change in those using moisturiser. The measurement of the barrier function of the skin showed an increase for three of the five moisturising products at day 7 and was sustained for one of the products at day 14. The authors concluded that regular application of moisturiser to normal skin offers a protective effect against repeated exposure to irritants, and may prevent the development of dermatitis in the healthcare environment.

Observational epidemiological studies

Case studies

Case studies are descriptions of individual cases of a disease or health issue. They provide a more indepth examination of factors which might cause a health effect, but do not indicate cause and effect. However they may highlight the need for further investigation and research. An example of a case study would be a case of dermatitis with exposure to a new chemical. If this was the first reported case, of itself it might not indicate a specific problem, but would flag up to healthcare workers to be vigilant in looking for further cases. In evidence reviews, case series may be taken into account, where several people with similar health issues are evaluated, for example, with an indication of how the disease has affected their ability to work.

Cohort studies (follow-up studies)

A cohort is a group of individuals sharing a common characteristic and observed over time in the group. This type of study compares two groups of people where one group is exposed to a hazard (e.g. noise, skin or respiratory sensitisers) and the other group is not exposed. Detailed records are made of the maximum and cumulative exposure and duration of employment. Ideally the groups will be similar with regard to gender and other social attributes. The presence of any disease which is associated with exposure is noted at follow-up in both the exposed and non-exposed group. A measure of the relative risk of the disease can be produced. The disadvantage of this type of study is that it requires considerable money, organisation and time.

COHORT STUDY EXAMPLE

Nielsen et al.[36] did a prospective study lasting 8.5 years on newly employed Swedish workers exposed to organic acid anhydrides (OAA) in three different factories. These substances are used as hardeners in epoxy resin systems and are powerful sensitisers, giving frequent rhinitis and asthma in exposed workers. The different factories used the OAA for the production of barrels for grenade firearms, to fix and isolate components in ignition systems and in the production of capacitors.

The individuals in the three groups were examined and had blood tests to detect sensitisation, on commencement and then every 1–2 years depending on the plant. The findings were that OAA exposure is associated with frequent symptoms of the eyes and airways in a dose–response-related manner. Symptoms appeared even at mean exposure levels as low as <10 $\mu g/m^3$. From this work an occupational exposure threshold level of <5 $\mu g/m^3$ was proposed. The study also found that smoking and atopy may affect the symptoms. Atopy involves the capacity to produce immunoglobulin E in response to common allergens, a genetic tendency to develop the classic allergic diseases – atopic dermatitis, allergic rhinitis (hayfever) and asthma.[37]

In historical cohort studies, data on exposure and health effect or disease are analysed retrospectively, for example, regarding occupational cancers. The data are already available at the start of the study and therefore this is a less costly form of research. It does rely on the accuracy of information on exposures such as job type, use of chemicals and environmental sampling data. It is useful if such information is routinely gathered and recorded to allow the identification of the individual many years later, using a unique identifier such as national insurance number.

HISTORICAL COHORT STUDY EXAMPLE

An example of this is a study undertaken of enzyme detergent worker by Cathcart et al.[38] In this UK study, the results of the respiratory health surveillance, including lung function testing, of 731 male workers from five locations were examined. Historical data were available for between 4 and 20 years, depending on the length of work. A calculation of exposure was made by looking at the job history. The rate of reduction of forced expiratory volume in 1 second and forced vital capacity, indicating onset of asthma, varied depending on the geographical location and by smoking habit. However there were no consistent trends with enzyme exposure.

Case control studies

In case control studies, 'cases' are persons who experience ill health from the disease under study and 'controls' are persons who are not ill, but are otherwise comparable to the cases, so have a similar lifestyle. When it is suspected that the disease is related to exposure to a hazard, a careful analysis is performed to establish to what extent persons in the case and control groups were exposed to the factors. If ill people are more often exposed than healthy people, then it may be concluded that there is a link between the health effect and the risk factor.

CASE CONTROL STUDY EXAMPLE

In the case control study that follows, the factors affecting the ability to return to work while experiencing back pain may be psychological. Brox et al.[39] looked at three groups with approximately 45 people in each. There were healthy controls, a group with short-term sickness absence due to subacute back pain and a group with chronic lower-back pain awaiting surgery. The groups were matched by age and gender. Measurements were made of disability, pain, psychological factors and physical performance. The results found that in the two patient groups there were comparable scores for self-rated working ability, fear avoidance beliefs for physical activity and aerobic capacity. There was a significant difference between the three groups in pain, emotional distress, and abdominal and back muscle endurance. Self-efficacy for pain and fear avoidance beliefs was measured using four questions, e.g. 'Do you believe you can reduce your symptoms by yourself?' and there was a significant difference between the two patient groups. The authors found a stepwise deterioration of pain, disability, psychological factors and physical performance from healthy controls to patients with chronic lower-back pain. It was suggested that interventions such as fear avoidance-based physiotherapy in the acute or subacute stage may be useful in reducing fear avoidance and promoting return to normal activity.

Cross-sectional studies

Cross-sectional studies, also known as prevalence studies, are restricted to a simple description of the frequency of new cases (incidence) and all existing cases (prevalence) and distribution of a disease within a population at a point in time. They may also be used in the regular recording of information such as health surveillance.

CROSS-SECTIONAL STUDY EXAMPLE

In 'Occupational asthma: a community based study' by de Bono and Hudsmith,[40] the general practice medical records of those who were known to have asthma in a South Oxfordshire practice were examined to see if any association was found with employment. The practice had 6,077 patients of working age, and of these, 346 (6 per cent) had a diagnosis of asthma. This was narrowed down to 182 with adult-onset asthma (53 per cent) and this group was the population that was studied. Of these, 157 (86 per cent) had at least one occupation recorded in their notes. Only one had had the occupation recorded at the time of diagnosis. Although approximately a third (32 per cent) were in jobs known to be significant causes of occupational asthma (e.g. nurses, bakers, animal workers, paint sprayers), the link between their occupation and symptoms had only been recorded in 18 per cent. The study also noted that 4 per cent of the patients with adult-onset asthma had been given a diagnosis of occupational asthma, although in the majority the diagnosis had not been confirmed by a specialist. The results suggest that a large number of adults with adult-onset asthma may have occupational exposures which might cause or contribute to their asthma. The opportunity to refer on to a respiratory specialist for diagnosis, and thus the possibility of avoiding the allergen, or to exclude the diagnosis, is being missed. This is also true of those for whom no occupation is being recorded. The authors concluded that educating GPs about occupational asthma and improving access to specialist advice would improve the situation.

A glossary for research in OH with about 20 specific concepts defined has been produced by Garcia and Checkoway.[41] This includes the 'healthy worker effect', acknowledging that those who are in employment are found to have better health than the general population, allowing them to undertake work, and manifesting as lower mortality rates. The 'healthy worker survivor effect' refers to the process by which those who find their health is affected by their work remove themselves from the activity by leaving, or transferring to less exposed jobs. Thus it appears that there is a lower risk in those who remain and this also causes challenges in dose–response estimation. This is of significance in cross-sectional studies of prevalence and exposure.

Evaluating research

Evaluating public health interventions can be a challenge as they can be complex. Clinical trials focus on eliminating potential confounding variables and usually involve highly motivated individuals with similar characteristics and who have no health conditions other than the one studied. This is not generally representative of the working population for whom OH practitioners provide advice. The outcomes of clinical trials may produce interventions that are expensive and demanding of the clients and health practitioners. These interventions may not transfer well into the community setting. It may be that low-intensity interventions which are less effective but can be delivered to larger numbers can have more impact.

Another aspect is that it may be that the apparent failure of an intervention has more to do with the appropriateness of the evaluation method rather than a problem with the intervention. If an intervention is unsuccessful, the evidence should help to determine whether there was a failure of intervention concept or theory, or if the intervention was just badly implemented.[42] The Health Development Agency created framework grading evidence and recommendations for public health interventions.[43] One model for examining research is the RE-AIM framework, which assesses five dimensions.[44] These are reach, efficacy, adoption, implementation and maintenance. The product of the five dimensions is the public health impact score.

Reach

Reach is a measure at the individual level (e.g. employee) of the percentage and risk characteristics of those who are affected by a policy or programme. It is the proportion of the target population that participated in the intervention. It also involves an understanding of the demographic information of the participant and of non-participants. The authors point out that those who participate in health promotion activities may be the 'worried well', likely to be more affluent and non-smokers. If there are small differences in risk levels between those participating and those not, because the interventions are scaled up to large numbers of people, there can be a significant impact on cost-effectiveness.

Efficacy

Efficacy is the success rate if implemented as in the guidelines. There are positive and negative outcomes to a health intervention. Positive outcomes are usually measured by an improvement in some targeted risk or health indicator. The negative effects can be the social and psychological effects of labelling a participant with a potential illness. The efficacy is defined as positive outcomes minus negative outcomes, ensuring that the benefits of the intervention outweigh the harm. Outcomes can be measured as biologic data (e.g. body mass index, lung function), but also as behavioural changes of the participants (e.g. smoking cessation), the staff (approaching patients and making follow-up calls) and of those who are paying for the invention by adopting it or changing policies. A patient-centred quality-of-life perspective should be included to allow evaluation of consumer satisfaction, functioning and mental wellbeing as these are a check on the impact of delivery practices.

Adoption

Adoption functions at an organisation level, and is an indication of the proportion of settings, such as workplaces, that adopt the intervention. This is usually measured by direct observation, interviews or surveys. If there are barriers to adoption, these should be assessed when evaluating settings which do not participate in the proposed intervention.

Implementation

Implementation is a measure of the extent to which the intervention is implemented as intended in the real world. Research interventions are undertaken in most studies by highly motivated researchers, whereas in the community they will be implemented by busy healthcare staff with many conflicting priorities, and may not be as successful.

Maintenance

Maintenance describes the long-term behaviour of the individual and the organisation with regard to the intervention. It is not uncommon for individuals who have changed health behaviours to relapse after a period of time. It is also important to check at the organisational level that the health promotion practice or policy has become routine and part of the everyday culture. Maintenance research may be required to document that policies continue to be implemented over time. It is suggested that this might be for 2 years or longer.

Undertaking research in the work environment

For those proposing to trial a health intervention themselves, the Medical Research Council has created a research evaluation framework (Box 9.1).[45] This is essential reading to give background to ensure that studies are well planned and the outcomes will be able to be implemented in the real world.[46]

Box 9.1   The development–evaluation–implementation process

Developing an intervention

- Are you clear about what you are trying to do: what outcome are you aiming for, and how will you bring about change?
- Does your intervention have a coherent theoretical basis?
- Have you used this theory systematically to develop the intervention?
- Can you describe the intervention fully, so that it can be implemented properly for the purposes of your evaluation and replicated by others?
- Does the existing evidence – ideally collated in a systematic review – suggest that it is likely to be effective or cost-effective?
- Can it be implemented in a research setting, and is it likely to be widely implementable if the results are favourable?

Piloting and feasibility

Questions to ask yourself include:

- Have you done enough piloting and feasibility work to be confident that the intervention can be delivered as intended?
- Can you make safe assumptions about effect sizes and variability, and rates of recruitment and retention in the main evaluation study?

Evaluating the intervention

- What design are you going to use, and why?
- Is an experimental design preferable and if so, is it feasible?
- If a conventional parallel-group randomised controlled trial is not possible, have you considered alternatives such as cluster randomisation or a stepped-wedge design?
- If the effects of the intervention are expected to be large or too rapid to be confused with secular trends, and selection biases are likely to be weak or absent, then an observational design may be appropriate.
- Have you set up procedures for monitoring delivery of the intervention, and overseeing the conduct of the evaluation?

Source: Medical Research Council (2008) Developing and evaluating complex interventions: New guidance. Available online at: www.mrc.ac.uk/complexinterventionsguidance.

It also gives details and examples of different types of experimental design more suited to public health, such as cluster randomised trials, stepped-wedge design and others for interventions where there might be ethical objections to withholding a potentially beneficial intervention to a group. These might be useful in the OH setting where there are plans to introduce a new process or intervention across several sites in an organisation.[47,48] It may be possible to gain useful information which can be more widely applied by careful consideration and documentation of the outcome of interventions which are part of existing business plans.

Conclusion

The participation in, and interpretation of, research is an essential tool for the OH nurse. There should be active and ongoing improvement in practice using the information gleaned from evidence-based guidance to ensure that clients receive the best possible advice and interventions.

References

1 Bonita R, Beaglehole R, Kjellström T (2006) *Basic Epidemiology*, 2nd edn. Available online at: http://whqlibdoc.who.int/publications/2006/9241547073_eng.pdf.

2 Franco G (1999) Ramazzini and workers' health. *Lancet* 354: September 4. Available online at: http://155.185.2.46/immagini4/lancet354_99_858.pdf.

3 Coggon D, Rose G, Barker DJP. *Epidemiology for the Uninitiated*, 4th edn. Available online at: http://www.bmj.com/about-bmj/resources-readers/publications/epidemiology-uninitiated.

4 United Kingdom Health Development Agency. *Getting Evidence into Practice in Public Health*. Available online at: http://www.nice.org.uk/niceMedia/documents/getting_eip_pubhealth.pdf.

5 Department of Health (2000) *The NHS Plan: A plan for investment, A plan for reform*. Available online at: http://www.dh.gov.uk/en/Publicationsandstatistics/Publications/PublicationsPolicyAndGuidance/DH_4002960.

6 Sacket DL, Rosenberg WM, Muir Gray JM, Haynes RB *et al.* (1996) Evidence based medicine, what it is and what it isn't. *Br Med J* 312: 71–72. Available online at: http://dx.doi.org/10.1136/bmj.312.7023.71.

7 Black N (1996) Why we need observational studies to evaluate the effectiveness of health care. *Br Med J* 12: 1215–1218. Available online at: http://dx.doi.org/10.1136/bmj.312.7040.1215.

8 Schaafsma F, Hulshol C, van Dijk F, Verbeek J (2004) Information demands of occupational health physicians and their attitude towards evidence-based methods. *Scand J Work Environ Hlth* 30 (4). Available online at: http://www.jstor.org/discover/10.2307/40968796?uid=3738032&uid=2&uid=4&sid=21101709968247.

9 Kelly MP, Chambers J, Huntley J, Millward L (2003) *Method 1 for the Production of Effective Action Briefings and Related Materials*. London: Health Development Agency. Available online at: http://www.nice.org.uk/aboutnice/whoweare/aboutthehda/evidencebase/keypapers/evidenceintopractice/evidence_into_practice_method_1_for_the_production_of_effective_action_briefings_and_related_materials.jsp.

10 British Occupational Health Research Foundation (2005, 2010) *Occupational Asthma – Identification, management and prevention: Evidence based review and guidelines*. Available online at: http://www.bohrf.org.uk/projects/asthma.html.

11 Nursing and Midwifery Council (2004) *Standards of Proficiency for Specialist Community Public Health Nurses*, p. 5. Available online at: http://www.nmc-uk.org/Documents/NMC-Publications/NMC-Standards-of-proficiency-for-specialist-communicty-public-health-nurses.pdf.

12 Faculty of Occupational Medicine (2010) *Occupational Health Service Standards for Accreditation*. Available online at: https://www.seqohs.org/DocumentStore/fom_seqohs.pdf p. 15 C2.4.

13 Alessio L, Crippa M, Porru S, Lucchini R, Placidi D, Vanoni O, Torri D (2006) From clinical activities to didactics and research in occupational medicine. *Med Lav* 97 (2): 393–401. Available online at: http://www.ncbi.nlm.nih.gov/pubmed/17017376.

14 http://www.nice.org.uk.

15 http://www.bohrf.org.uk.

16 http://www.hse.gov.uk.

17 http://www.nhshealthatwork.co.uk/evidence-based-guidelines.asp.

18 http://www.rcplondon.ac.uk/rcp/clinical-standards-department/health-and-work-development-unit.

19 http://www.rcn.org.uk/development/library/elibrary.

20 Royal College of Nursing databases. Available online at: http://www.rcn.org.uk/development/library/elibrary/databases_to_search.

21 Royal Society of Medicine databases. Available online at: http://www.rsm.ac.uk/librar/cddatabase.php.

22 Nicholson P (2007) How to undertake a systematic review in an occupational setting. *Occup Environ Med* 64 (5): 353–358. Available online at: http://www.ncbi.nlm.nih.gov/pmc/articles/PMC2092548.

23 Verbeek J, Salmi J, Pasternak I, Jauhiainen M (2005) A search strategy for occupational health intervention studies. *Occup Environ Med* 62: 682–687. Available online at: http://oem.bmj.com/content/62/10/682.abstract.

24 http://www.bmj.com/about-bmj/resources-readers/publications/how-read-paper.

25 Greenhalgh T (1997) How to read a paper: Statistics for the non-statistician. I: Different types of data need different statistical tests. *BMJ* 315: 364. Available online at: http://www.bmj.com/content/315/7104/364.

26 Greenhalgh T (1997) How to read a paper: Statistics for the non-statistician. II: 'Significant' relations and their pitfalls. *BMJ* 315: 422. Available online at: http://dx.doi.org/10.1136/bmj.315.7105.422.

27 Hoe J, Hoare Z (2012) Understanding quantitative research part 1. *Nurs Stand* 27 (15–17): 52–57. Available online at: http://nursingstandard.rcnpublishing.co.uk/archive/article-understanding-quantitative-research-part-one.

28 Hoe J, Hoare Z (2012) Understanding quantitative research part 2. *Nurs Stand* 27 (18): 348–355. Available online at: http://nursingstandard.rcnpublishing.co.uk/archive/article-understanding-quantitative-research-part-2.

29 Rowntree D (2000) *Statistics Without Tears: A primer for non-mathematicians.* London: Penguin.

30 The Pennsylvania State University (2012) *Online Course 507: Epidemiological research methods. Lessons.* Available online at: https://onlinecourses.science.psu.edu/stat507/01/intro.

31 Sorohan TM (1995) *An Introduction to Medical Statistics.* Course notes M Med Sc(Occ Health), University of Birmingham.

32 http://www.diabetes.co.uk/diabetes_care/blood-sugar-level-ranges.html.

33 http://www.mathsisfun.com/data/standard-normal-distribution.html.

34 Röhrig B, du Prel JB, Wachtlin D, Blettner M (2009) Types of study in medical research. *Dtsch Arztebl Int* 106 (15): 262–268. Available online at: 10.3238/arztebl.2009.0262.

35 Williams C, Wilkinson SM, McShane P, Lewis J, Pennington D, Pierce S, Fernandez C (2010) A double-blind, randomized study to assess the effectiveness of different moisturizers in preventing dermatitis induced by hand washing to simulate healthcare use. *Br J Dermatol* 162 (5): 1088–1092. Available online at: http://www.ncbi.nlm.nih.gov/pubmed/20199550.

36 Nielsen J, Welinder H, Bessyrd I, Rylander L (2006) Ocular and airway symptoms related to organic acid anhydride exposure – a prospective study. *Allergy* 61 (6): 743–749. Available online at: http://onlinelibrary.wiley.com/doi/10.1111/j.1398-9995.2006.01028.x/full.

37 http://www.medterms.com.

38 Cathcart M, Nicholson D, Roberts D, Bazley M *et al.* (1997) Enzyme exposure, smoking and lung function in employees in the detergent industry over 20 years. *Occup Med* 47 (8): 473–478. Available online at: http://occmed.oxfordjournals.org/content/47/8/473.short.

39 Brox J, Storheim K, Holm I, Friis A, Reikera O (2005) Disability, pain, psychological factors and physical performance in healthy controls, patients with sub-acute and chronic low back pain: A case-control study. *J Rehabil Med* 37: 95–99. Also see *European*

Guidelines for the Management of Chronic Non-Specific Low Back Pain, November 2004. Available online at: http://www.backpaineurope.org/web/files/WG2_Guidelines. pdf.

40 de Bono J, Hudsmith L (1999) Occupational asthma: A community based study. *Occup Med* 49 (4): 217–219. Available online at: http://occmed.oxfordjournals.org/content/49/4/217. full.pdf.

41 Garcia A, Checkoway H (2003) A glossary for research in occupational health. *J Epidemiol Commun Hlth* 57: 7–10. Available online at: http://jech.bmj.com/content/ 57/1/7.full.

42 Rychetnik L, Frommer M, Hawe P, Sheill A (2002) Criteria for evaluating evidence in public health interventions. *J Epidemiol Commun Hlth* 56: 119–127. Available online at: jech.bmj.com/content/56/2/119.

43 Weightman A, Ellis S, Cullum A, Sander L, Turley R (2005) *Grading Evidence and Recommendations for Public Health Interventions: Developing and piloting a framework Health Development Agency.* Available online at: http://www.nice.org.uk/nicemedia/ docs/grading_evidence.pdf.

44 Glasgow R, Vogt T, Boles S (1999) Evaluating the public health impact of health promotion interventions: The RE-AIM framework. *Am J Public Hlth* 89 (9): 1322–1327. Available online at: http://www.ncbi.nlm.nih.gov/pubmed/10474547.

45 Medical Research Council (2008) *Developing and Evaluating Complex Interventions: New guidance.* Available online at: www.mrc.ac.uk/complexinterventionsguidance.

46 Craig P, Dieppe P, Macintyre S, Mitchie S *et al.* (2008) Developing and evaluating complex interventions: The new Medical Research Council guidance. *BMJ* 33: a1655. Available online at: http://www.ncbi.nlm.nih.gov/pmc/articles/PMC2769032.

47 Stone S, Slade R, Fuller C, Charlett A, Cookson B, Teare L, *et al.* (2007) Early communication: Does a national campaign to improve hand hygiene in the NHS work? Initial English and Welsh experience from the NOSEC study (National Observational Study to Evaluate the CleanYourHands Campaign). *J Hosp Infect* 66 (3): 293–296. Available online at: http://www.biomedcentral.com/1753-6561/5/S6/P117.

48 National Patient Safety Agency (2010) *Stopping Infection in Its Tracks.* Available online at: www.npsa.nhs.uk/EasySiteWeb/GatewayLink.aspx?allId=73513.

10 Quality and audit in occupational health

Sarah Mogford

Learning objectives

After reading this chapter you will be able to:

- differentiate between quality and audit, whilst appreciating their interdependence
- appreciate the relevance of audit in the occupational health (OH) setting and professional practice
- be aware of existing standards, specific regulatory requirements and individual professional standards
- discuss the audit process and its significance and limitations in maintaining and raising standards in OH practice.

Purpose and scope

The topic of quality and audit is complex and covers the clinical, service delivery and business aspects of OH. The purpose of this chapter is to outline the differences between 'quality' and 'audit', how they interrelate and their significance in the OH context. It is not possible to cover comprehensively so vast a subject within this chapter alone; however, it will give an understanding of the overall subject and signpost to further sources.

There is great diversity between OH settings, together with the competing internal and external business, professional and statutory constraints. It is therefore not possible to set out any formal guidance for either individual OH practitioners or organisations on 'how to' audit their organisation and practice. The scope of this chapter is to give readers the tools to appreciate and assess any existing audit provision for its effectiveness and to signpost them to further information and resources to adapt for their own specific requirements.

Context

Quality service provision is increasingly important within individual organisations and the purchasers/users of their products and services. Individual professions are developing and incorporating audit as a tool to ensure that their members meet stated professional standards. Improving the quality of health service provision has been a high priority of government and social policy within the UK for many years. However, until the Black report,[1] most of the focus had been on hospital and (more recently) general practitioner and primary care trust services despite international drivers, such as the World Health Organization,[2] specifically targeting European OH audit over a decade ago. The importance of using audit for improving the quality of healthcare services has long been recognised.[3,4,5] As the Black report firmly put emphasis on setting and raising the standards and quality of OH provision in the UK, the importance of OH professionals having a sound understanding of quality and audit within their own professional practice and service provision is paramount.

Definition of terms

The terms quality and audit, whilst having discrete meanings, are often used interchangeably or with other terms in relation to assessing or measuring standards.

Quality

Quality is arguably a term that has different meanings to different people and within different contexts. The philosophical debate on quality definition can be summarised by Pursig,[6] who stated that quality could not be defined, but that individuals recognised quality when they encountered it. However, the various definitions within business and service settings do have similar threads:

- Quality involves meeting or exceeding customer expectations.
- Quality applies to products, services, people, processes, environment and education.
- Quality is an ever-changing concept or state – what is considered as quality today may not meet expectations tomorrow.

Many services and products claim 'quality' without any tangible proof and it is a term with some implied social and cultural meaning. Yet 'quality' is strived for by both the consumer and provider and is a frequently quoted aim in professional standards. Therefore, the importance of defining exactly what is meant by 'quality' when defining standards or striving to improve the quality of services is imperative to success.

Any feature or necessity of a service that is required for it to meet consumer or customer needs is often termed a 'quality characteristic'. Again, as with most concepts dealing with quality, the key is defining these accurately within the specific service delivered and having an effective way of measuring their delivery. This enables them to be defined in contracts for managing internal and external department expectations and therefore managing quality of service throughout (Table 10.1).

Table 10.1 Examples of service quality characteristics

Accessibility	Credibility	Integrity
Accuracy	Dependability	Promptness
Comfort	Effectiveness	Reliability
Competence	Efficiency	Responsiveness
Courtesy	Flexibility	Security

Source: Hoyle D (2007) *Quality Management Essentials*. Oxford: Butterworth-Heinemann, p. 16.

Activity

Pick two of the service quality characteristics from Table 10.1. Consider how they are relevant in the OH service or your individual practice. Are there any differences in their relevance/importance to service users, employees, managers, provision partners? How could you define them for OH service delivery and how could this be measured (i.e. audited)?

Note: you will review this 'measurement' later in the chapter.

Audit

Audit appears to be a less nebulous concept than quality, with a plethora of competing tools and methodology available to undertake the process. There are whole specialisms dealing with financial audit, audit management and clinical audit. Although arguably having more tangible meaning than quality, the concept of audit is nonetheless complex. It has its own conflicts with regard to methodology and scope within varying contexts.

Audit can be a tool for improving practice, care or services provided. As a basic audit, it is used to measure current practice and services provided against a set of standards or criteria. One weakness is that this can become a meaningless 'tick box' exercise when evidence is just sought to ensure standards are met – and a wasted exercise if the standards or methods used to assess them do not relate to practice. Hence audit is only as good as the standards/criteria the actual performance is measured against, and the skill of the individuals undertaking the audit. The *audit process* or *quality audit* goes further; it is used to identify areas of improvement and make necessary changes to practice. The NHS introduced 'clinical audit' in the 1989 Working for Patients initiative[7] (as opposed to the optional 'medical audit' that predated this). The aim of this was to use a quality improvement process to improve patient care, with an audit cycle being one of the driving tools. One of the main definers of clinical audit is that structure and outcome of care are collected and measured against very specific criteria. A main aspect of this process was the emphasis on drivers for change and quality improvement.

Audit is one way of measuring quality, as defined by standards measured, and a quality audit can be likened to an evaluation process.

Shaw[8] defines effective healthcare audit as having three elements: 'agreed criteria for "good" practice; methods of measuring against these criteria; and mechanisms for implementing appropriate change in practice.' This is very similar to the NHS clinical audit ethos. The *Oxford Dictionary*[9] defines audit as a noun and a verb: 'a systematic review or assessment of something.' However, a comprehensive definition of the verb comes from a non-business and non-financial source[10]: 'Auditing is the systematic examination of an entity, such as an organisation, facility or site, to determine whether, and to what extent, it conforms to specified standards.'

Quality audits or audit cycles are performed to verify conformance with standards through review of objective evidence. For best benefits, they should report where standards are not met and recommend areas for improvement, as well as highlighting and benchmarking areas of excellence to allow information sharing, thus developing bodies of expertise and practice that enhance continual improvement (Figure 10.1). As some professionals' OH activity will fall within the NHS remit, and professional OH activity involves aspects of clinical practice, for the purposes of this chapter 'clinical audit' will not be treated as a separate activity, but included in the universal definition.

So having established a clearer idea of what audit is, it remains to consider:

1. What is to be audited? What are the standards?
2. How/what methods to use in audit?
3. Who undertakes the audit and when?

It is important to get the above right and appropriate and to ensure that the results are 'reliable' and 'consistent'.

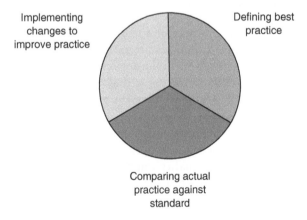

Figure 10.1 Outline audit cycle

For the purposes of OH professional individual and organisational practice, to meet the recommendations in the Black report, any auditing needs to be that of an audit process or quality audit rather than a 'tick box' approach (Figure 10.1).

Activity

Audit = a structured performance review against agreed standards

Quality = the extent that performance meets the agreed standards

Consider how far these two definitions cover the activity of measuring performance in the OH setting. What else would you add? What limiting factors need to be considered?

Relevance in occupational health setting

Auditing quality in nursing practice has been of concern since the beginning of modern nursing when Florence Nightingale called for systematic collection and analysis of data and identification of practice standards.[11] In contemporary occupational settings, along with recent political drivers following the Black report, the impetus for quality audits has been from managing costs whilst improving standards and meeting statutory and regulatory standards. Another important aspect is establishing any gaps in evidence-based standards which should then generate research. A simple audit system that checks procedures in place can be invaluable in identifying potential problems or loopholes in processes and compliance with legislative requirements. If undertaken on a regular basis, it is an ideal time to check that procedures are up to date and to review in light of performance and changing needs. Although audit is often used as a tool for root cause analysis for profession and management problems, prevention is better than cure.

As OH is very much a business offering a service for other businesses, their management concepts apply. Arguably, in the UK, this has been far more than other traditional healthcare provision as, up to 2013 at least, OH is not an NHS (i.e. state-funded) function, but reliant on employer provision and funding. The establishment of state-funded access to OH assessment is being trialled at the time of writing and recommended in the Department for Work and Pensions fit note advice for employers[12] – how successful its implementation and potential impact are remain to be seen.[13] Audit is an essential tool within OH to facilitate the justification of the value of its function to existing and potential clients. The historical status of OH within the UK does leave it vulnerable to being high in the perceived 'non-essential' services to be cut when reducing costs in challenging economic climates. OH can be seen as 'non-essential' in the business world, so using an effective audit to prove the value and cost-effectiveness of the service is often essential to the survival of the service in the competing service sector. If the audit proves and adds quality of service, this can not only be a key selling point, but also a motivator for professionals involved. It can therefore be argued that OH needs to step up to the mark and prioritise audit, as does the pure business world in which it operates. In the world of business, audit results are initiated and used at the highest levels. In manufacturing process, audit is an essential tool to review methods and check compliance (see Example 10.1, where audit found the flaw in the process that affected both costs and quality). When used effectively, as demonstrated in the example, it can make the difference between a failing and a successful business in terms of costs and quality.

The two drivers of professional clinical standards and business effectiveness that exist in OH are equally prioritised, though possibly with different motivations for audit of quality.

The increasing use of litigation in modern society can also be an argument for the use of audit – although one would hope from a professional perspective that this was a secondary rather than primary motivation. Having quantifiable results of tested and consistent procedures and results can be useful in many contexts; defence in litigation is just one of them (Example 10.1).

Example 10.1 Manufacture example of audit cutting costs

After a failing business, Fairline (boat manufacturer) had been acquired, an audit identified much wastage and error (poor quality) in the method of wiring. The existing system allowed for each piece of wire to be cut and wired individually, thus leaving room for wasted resources, including time, error and customer dissatisfaction. The introduction of a new technique (wiring harness) standardised the process, improving quality whilst reducing waste and labour time and increasing customer satisfaction.

Source: Jon Moulton (Director) Becap GP Ltd, quoted from BBC 'Bottom Line' interview October 2012, discussing the importance of audit.

Challenge specific to OH

OH varies greatly in how it is provided, including from sole independent practitioners to in-house provision (which may or may not also sell OH services to others) to large international healthcare providers and the NHS. There is an emerging provision for a state-funded free-access service linked to sickness absence, currently under trial. OH can operate in a variety of settings, often highly specialised with very specific agendas and operating procedures.

Therefore standards that may be applicable in one OH setting may not apply in another. Standard operating procedures within a single OH provider may even vary from client to client. The chain of management control can also be very complex, with internal OH department management structures, in addition to the overall operating or parent company controls, working partners such as human resources, health and safety, psychological service partners and other clinical specialities. This is in addition to client needs. Even identifying the client within an OH setting is fraught with complexity and competing needs and expectations. The client can range from individual employees who have the appointment, their manager who has referred them, the department who is paying the invoice and any regulatory bodies that need reporting to. All of these will have some form of contact/communication with the OH professional and levels of expectation and service delivery.

Therefore, finding one system to apply to all OH service providers that is comprehensive, but flexible enough to account for the differences, is a monumental task. For many OH businesses, choosing an external quality system, or validating an internal one, is driven by tender or business requirements. This may lead to a system being in place that is not necessarily the best tool for the individual OH service due to external factors beyond their control.

Any audit system needs to cover all aspects of OH function. Within OH, the basic areas of distinct function include:

- the professional OH clinical service (including education)
- the business/administration of running an OH service
- meeting client needs
- financial control
- meeting statutory and regulatory control
- identifying gaps in service and areas of change.

These may overlap and often (for example, with client needs) have areas of potential conflict. Hence the importance of having clear and accurate standards or protocols to ensure everyone involved, from OH professional to commissioning client and service user, has clear expectations. Figure 10.2 shows a simplified breakdown of areas within OH that should be considered for a quality audit.

Structure

Structure can include the provision of staff numbers and their qualifications in addition to any physical environment in which OH activity takes place. It can also include stored data and record keeping. These areas are largely dictated by legislative requirements and are measures of results (often tick box). Although essential to measure compliance, they do not necessarily indicate any measure of service being performed. A superb facility, with compliant records and good staffing levels, does not guarantee good, effective and relevant OH advice to the client.

Process

Process can include the administrative process that underlies all OH activity and communication, the risk assessments on which the basis of much OH activity is based and clinical activity and training. As much of this process is paramount to the meeting of

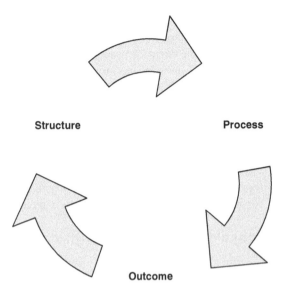

Structure

Process

Outcome

Figure 10.2 Occupational health audit: basic areas

client and professional clinical standard needs, ensuring standards are appropriate and measuring them in a meaningful way is important for quality of service delivery.

Outcome

There are varied ways of looking at outcome within OH using result and performance audits. Improvement in sickness absence levels and early return to work can be specific to industry or extended to a broader environment (often compared between public and private sector). National targets are one driver of audit of outcome and often involve external reporting and are under regulatory control. Drivers specific to OH providers can include client (at all levels) satisfaction surveys, feedback meetings and meeting time targets and may overlap with structure and process in content.

Standard setting: results/outcome versus performance – which are being measured?

When designing standards against which to measure (audit), for an effective system, it is important that these standards are appropriate. One essential part of this is understanding the difference between measuring result (outcome) and performance. Both of these have relevance in OH. One simple analogy of the difference is looking at the measure of a car speedometer reading. The reading shown on a car speedometer is a result. A measure of performance could be the fuel consumption or the car engine temperature if auditing the engine efficiency. Alternatively, a measure of performance could be the way the car is driven on the road or distance between vehicles if auditing

Table 10.2   Basic differences between result and
performance measures/indicators

Result (outcome)	Performance
Can be financial or non-financial, e.g. costs or results of customer surveys	Non-financial measures
Measures usually longer-term, e.g. monthly, quarterly	Measured regularly, e.g. 24/7, daily, weekly
Cannot be tied to discrete activity	Tied to discrete activity, thus to team or individual, and allows responsibility
Result of more than one activity, therefore poor indicator of where specific intervention needed or specific progress made	As tied to specific activity, easier to identify what is required to sustain or improve results

Source: adapted from Parmenter D (2012) *Key Performance Indicators: Developing, implementing and using winning KPIs*, 2nd edn. John Wiley, p. 10.

driver efficiency. Table 10.2 shows the basic differences between result and performance measures/indicators.

In auditing, as with research, ensuring that the correct tool is used to measure is essential to success. Both quantitative and qualitative measures are valid in the appropriate setting. Audit can be retrospective, descriptive and analytical. It can include random sampling (and, as with research, what is random?), surveys and documentation reviews.

The motivation for audit can be complex and multifaceted. However, it is important to establish (as far as practicable) the main drivers and the audience for results. For example, is the audit to satisfy the auditing body? Is obtaining an external award and so satisfying those standards the main purpose? Is the purpose to serve evidence to the customer, the employees, the OH provider or meeting targets for statutory or business drivers? Establishing this and prioritising are necessary – it is impractical and unrealistic to audit all aspects of OH service. Establishing this can also serve to define any gaps when using an 'off-the-peg' or external auditing service that may have to be used for reasons previously discussed. Identifying gaps or additional audit requirements of the individual service and developing a system of undertaking this independently may be the way to ensure the process is effective and meaningful (Example 10.2).

Activity

Revisit the first activity in this chapter and the methods you considered for measuring service quality characteristics. Do these methods measure result (outcome) or performance? Would you consider changing/adapting your original method considered and how?

Example 10.2   External versus internal audit: result versus performance

In an example cited by Agius,[14] a business had passed its ISO 9000 audit, including assessment of the business's occupational health (OH) department. However, when the OH department was audited by OH physicians as part of a peer review system, deficits were found in the respiratory health surveillance process. These deficits were that the questionnaire used was not one that was validated (evidence suggests that appropriate questionnaire assessment is a more accurate tool for predicting occupational asthma than lung function testing). Deficiencies were also found in assessing exposure to risk at source and methods of determining which employees required health surveillance. This therefore questioned the basis on which the whole process of the surveillance programme was based.

The ISO audit had been satisfied, so to all intents and purposes the OH unit had met the standards set – that it had a health surveillance programme, that the equipment was correct, maintained and calibrated, and appropriately qualified staff were used. The ISO assessed outcome or result – that processes were in place or actions had been taken. The peer review had looked at the performance – the methods and processes in place for obtaining these results.

Principles and benefits for quality standards (benchmarking)

Improving quality is important at every level:

- It maintains/increases customer base by giving customers the service they want/expect.
- It facilitates business success by delivering effective, efficient services.
- Quantifiable evidence with regard to performance is obtained.
- Quality increases job satisfaction through meeting the human need for a sense of accomplishment and professionalism.

Benchmarking or collecting data can help develop standards and is especially useful in areas where no definitive standards exist. It is one way of facilitating the establishment of relevant and appropriate standards against which to measure. It is also a way of increasing and enhancing professional standards and increasing the body of OH-specific evidence-based practice that was highlighted as lacking in the Black report.[1]

Benchmarking – sharing best practice – can be undertaken at local and national level. Peer support and multidisciplinary cross-professional working can only enhance this.

In addition to the National Institute for Health and Care Excellence (NICE),[15] the NHS has developed the Management of Health at Work Knowledge or MoHAWK,[16] which has also developed quality benchmarking criteria for OH. Stage 2 of the process invites OH providers from all sectors to share good practice and (at the time of writing) is a free service with 6-monthly data collection periods. The Association of Occupational Health Nurse Practitioners (UK) (AOHNP (UK)),[17] along with other professional organisations, has benchmarking as one of its core activities with the aim of raising standards. The British Occupational Health Research Foundation[18] is also a source of evidence-based material and guidance.

Statutory and professional standards for quality and audit in occupational health

These are often set at national policy level and are outside the individual OH service's or practitioners' control. However the standards may form the basis of OH delivery and therefore standards for audit. Professional bodies and regulation controls not only set the need for audit within the OH setting, but some also set standards to audit against. Many of the clinical functions either have some form of statutory regulation (e.g. in the UK, health surveillance under Control of Substances Hazardous to Health) or professional best-practice guidelines. At the very basic level, OH nursing advisers are required to audit that their practice and care are of a high standard (i.e. of quality) to meet their professional obligation in the Nursing and Midwifery Council (NMC) Code of Conduct.[19] Amongst other matters, the code details 13–17 specifics regarding obtaining consent and 42–47 with record keeping. Chapter 1 of this book details the NMC standards for the specialist practitioner role, which include 'developing quality and risk management with an evaluative culture'.

However, enforcement is often reliant on the individual practitioner or provider. The Faculty of Occupational Medicine (FOM) has undertaken work in the field of establishing tools to assess career OH physicians and trainees and to assist in the revalidation process.[20] Agius developed the Correspondence Assessment/Audit Tool in/for Occupational Health (CATOH) following the finding that referrals for sickness absence, and therefore the correspondence for such, constituted the bulk of the work of Members and Fellows of the Faculty. CATOH is a tool that can be used to audit both outcome and process of any correspondence, assessing quality[14,21,22,23] (Table 10.3). It is also an example of an audit tool that is continually under its own audit process and adapts to feedback. It has been established and supported by research-based evidence. It takes factors such as confidentiality into consideration and is possibly a tool (based on research originally supported by FOM) that could be adapted for other than OH physicians' correspondence.

Activity

Take a report that either you have written, or an OH report you have access to. Using the CATOH tool and concentrating on the formative assessment section, assess the contents. Reflect on any improvements to the report, and the scope of the CATOH tool.

**Table 10.3   Version 2B of Correspondence Assessment/
Audit Tool in/for Occupational Health (CATOH)**

Name of physician being audited/trainee being assessed or else any confidential
   identifying number:

Name of auditing physician/trainee's assessor:

Date of assessment

Other relevant information, e.g. OHS, clinic etc.:

Mode of selection of letter (please tick, circle, or underline one):

A. Chosen by trainee/physician being audited/assessed

B. Chosen by assessor/auditor

C. Random

How?

(e.g. Specify sampling frame: time interval, etc.)

Reference and provenance of letter:

Reference number:

Date of letter:

Is it a follow-up letter?

(Please do not include any patient/subject identifier)

Nature of addressee (please tick, circle, or underline one):

Manager ('line' or HR):

Other doctor:

Copied to patient? :

Other (please specify):

Nature of original referral (please tick, circle, or underline one):

Management

Self

Routine health surveillance

Pre-employment

Other (please specify)

Note: If this is part of a wider audit other information might need to
   be recorded, e.g.:

Date of receipt of letter of referral:

Date of first appointment offered to patient/worker:

Date of consultation:

Date of letter:

Compliance (if applicable) with any explicit consent policy:

Other (local) adaptations:

Items to be considered for the purposes of the audit/formative assessment:
1. Is the nature and reason for the referral determining the letter clear?
2. Is the workplace, occupation and occupational context, i.e. relevant exposures/ work demands of the patient, specified?
3. Is there a clear and valid statement of current fitness for work?
4. Are all the domains (of attendance, performance and safety) where relevant to health issues adequately addressed?
5. Is there a clear and valid statement of the likely date of return to work?
6. Is there a clear and valid statement of future degree of fitness for work or residual disability?
7. Is there a clear and valid statement on whether work could be affecting/have affected the patient's health?
8. Are there clear and valid rehabilitation (or workplace adjustment) recommendation(s)?
9. Is there evidence of an explicit response to any other appropriate patient's or referring manager's question(s) being answered? (e.g. about DDA)
10. Is there reference to an appropriate patient follow-up plan?
11. Is there reference to an appropriate past or future workplace assessment?
12. Is there evidence of the letter being copied to or its content shared with the patient?
13. Is other significant information omitted?
14. Is there irrelevant (or indiscreet) information?
15. Is the letter well structured and clear to understand?

Feedback on version 2B of CATOH:
Name of respondent (optional but preferable):
Status: Trained occupational physician/trainee/other (please specify)
Date:

Feedback based on perusing the document (not necessarily applying it)
Do you agree that as far as appropriate and feasible the same tool should be used both for purposes of audit and for formative assessment of trainees?
Yes/No/Don't know
Any other comments on the 'rationale' or on CATOH itself:

Feedback based on using CATOH:
Did you use CATOH as an audit tool?   Yes/No
If yes: How many physicians were involved?
        How many letters/reports were audited?
Did you use CATOH as a formative assessment tool for trainees? Yes/No
If yes: How many trained physicians were involved?
        How many trainees were involved?
        How many letters/reports were audited?

(continued)

Table 10.3 (Continued)

Feedback on the specific CATOH questions:

Please provide any specific feedback you wish on the 15 CATOH questions below, citing the relevant question number.

In particular please state whether you feel that any of the questions are likely to be redundant in most cases, and should therefore be removed. Please give reasons if you can. (This will be helpful in simplifying CATOH.)

OHS, occupational health service; HR, human resources; DDA, Disability Discrimination Act.

Source: Agius R (undated) *Correspondence Assessment/Audit Tool in/for Occupational Health (CATOH)*. Available online at: www.agius.com/hew/audit/catoh.htm.

Example 10.2 demonstrated a potential difference between internal and external auditing. However, many professional and regulatory standards share the problem that it is so often outcome (or that something exists or has been done) rather than the detail of the process that is measured.

External quality awards, industry standards

Many large organisations, or those with very specific functions, may have their own industry standards that are then applied to their OH providers (be they in-house or external providers). Smaller organisations may well internally audit that they meet the professional and regulatory requirements and have their own quality checks for these and other activities. However, there is a huge industry in itself that is dedicated to providing external quality awards. As already discussed, the rationale for using an external quality award may be to meet tender/business requirements as opposed to specific quality drivers. Embarking on standard setting and establishing an effective audit system from scratch can be a daunting task. It may be preferable and more cost-effective in terms of time (though any audit process, internal or external, is very consuming of the commodity of time) to meet the fees of an external provider, many of whom are fee paying. Certainly, having demonstrated that you have met a known and recognised standard can not only be a morale boost to the receiving business, but of commercial worth. The quality and audit management business has a voluntary regulatory body – the Chartered Quality Institute (CQI) – and most reputable external providers such as ISO are registered with the CQI.

The FOM with stakeholders devised the Safe Effective Quality Occupational Health Services (SEQOHS)[24] and has attempted to provide a national quality system for all OH providers. The NHS has committed to accredit its OH provision with this system, which uses auditors from within the 'recognised' OH environment. It also has the advantage of allowing existing ISO accreditation to be accepted for relevant criteria, thus negating the need to duplicate audit, but still having to pay both award bodies. As SEQOHS standards are in the public domain, they can be used or adapted internally without necessarily committing to the full SEQOHS audit system and fee paying – thus it is another benchmark. Whilst undoubtedly a huge step forward, and a tool that can be used, it has not been without criticism. This has included the type and process of

Table 10.4 Safe Effective Quality Occupational Health Services (SEQOHS): six domain standard groupings

1. Business probity (business integrity and financial propriety)
2. Information governance (adequacy and confidentiality of records)
3. People (competency and supervision of occupational health staff)
4. Facilities and equipment (safe, accessible and appropriate)
5. Relationships with purchasers (fair dealing and customer focus)
6. Relationship with workers (fair treatment, respect and involvement)

audit, the lack of independent or external appeals process, the FOM drivers for this audit system (predating Black) and indeed the auditors themselves. However, this is a relatively new quality system and one that should develop over time.

This leads on to the topic of ethics within audit and motivation of both the audit process and those undertaking it. Confidentiality of data is particularly relevant within OH and, when considering audit (auditors, access to and publishing of data), this has to be considered from commercial sensitivity, clinical files, personal data and confidentiality. When using medical or personal files for audit or research, it is essential that consent for this extends to those accessing information. Many contracts of employment contain a clause covering this and it is a consideration when using auditors whose primary role – and thus confidentiality remit – is not within the specific OH setting. Any bias of auditors (internal or external fee paying) needs to be considered, as an auditor with specific interests needs to be thoroughly understood when interpreting results. Revisiting professional codes of conduct and the statutory duties with regard to data protection and human rights and reflecting on this is a useful exercise when considering such issues (Table 10.4).

Limitations, change process and unexpected impact of audit

Limitations of an inappropriate or ineffective audit system have already been mentioned earlier in the chapter. Part of an effective audit system is having systems in place to acknowledge and deal with any unexpected impact of the audit process. This includes the potential need to change in light of audit findings.

Establishing and carrying out an effective audit process to improve quality within OH is difficult, even just as an academic or theoretical exercise. In reality, with all the competing aspects within the OH environment, what should work in theory may have an unexpected outcome in practice. A typical unexpected outcome includes overprioritising audit process, thus during audit process, there is a reduction in main OH function with reduced productivity. This does register on the audit, but only after a period of time, during which there can be dissatisfaction from the purchasing client, amongst others. This could be prevented by an effective preplanning process, but in reality there will be factors that are not anticipated. Although continual improvement and best practice are always aims, resources and competing business need may be a limiting factor.

Table 10.5   Examples of factors influencing resistance to audit process and change

Vested interests

Routines and habits

Risk of error/fear of failure/stress and anxiety re process

Conflict with personal goals

Threats to employees':
    role
    economic/job security
    self-esteem
    social networks/workplace relationships

Work load (actual or perceived)

Conflict with audit process or auditors

Existing workplace/organisational culture

In any area that deals with people, there is also the human factor to consider. The audit process does involve examining individual practice, behaviour and change. Individuals involved may be very anxious, even stressed by the process. A skilled auditor with an effective method (and using continual audit cycle) should be able to detect whether a result is a 'one-off' undertaken to meet the standard being measured, or part of everyday/regular activity. That is, standards are consistent and reliable over time. The human response to examination and change can be complex and not always positive and factors, described in Table 10.5, need to be taken into account.

As the audit cycle is a continuous process and fluid, flexible and not fixed, this should allow early review of any problems encountered and necessary adaptations to process to be made. However, this relies on the skill of those undertaking the audit process and their motivation. Auditors, or an organisation whose motivation is 'we just want to survive this audit process', are unlikely to succeed in improving quality. Although the organisation may pass the audit (depending on what is measured), it is unlikely to have consistent results. Motivation which stems from the desire to maintain and improve performance and service is more likely to engage with a thorough audit process and succeed in its aims.

What and how to start the audit cycle in OH service/practice?

It is seen that all professionals working within OH, by definition of the need to maintain registration with their professional body and practice within statutory and regulatory remits, are undertaking some form of audit of their activities. This may just be of their clinical/professional practice. Is this enough? Professional and business drivers obviously argue not – and it would be concerning to find anyone operating within society's litigation and commercial drivers who could not see the relevance and importance of audit and the application of results in many arenas. Oakley[25] discusses the additional benefits of establishing an effective quality and audit process when undertaking any new OH contract. The audit process facilitates the logical thinking, prioritising and consultation that are essential for assuring good standards across practice and business areas of OH. An important point is that the inability 'to demonstrate a quality service costs money'. This is not only in terms of lost/dissatisfied customers, but inefficient use of resources (as seen in Example 10.1) and retention of staff. Although the benefits of audit may be slow in showing evidence in the wider clinical aspects of OH (morbidity, mortality and sickness absence), it may be seen more readily within the business and administration side of OH practice.

It could be easy to forget that the primary function of OH is not audit, but provision of services. An individual OH unit therefore needs to find the balance in its allocation of resources, in how much to allocate to the audit process. Considering what needs to be audited is also important – is there value in auditing every process? The preplanning of audit process and clarity of what you are aiming to achieve from each criterion measured may be time consuming, but so often is time well spent. Deciding what, how, how often and who undertakes audit is very much an individual business decision.

Many OH units start with ensuring professional and statutory standards along with meeting any existing 'primary business' quality audits. Then they undertake a 'gap' analysis and establish additional standards specific to their environment. If this had been undertaken in the business quoted in Example 10.2, specific OH procedures might have been checked so the peer review would also have passed the OH unit.

Customers may have their own quality standards to meet that influence the choice or scope of OH audit tool or processes in addition to standards. As there is so much variance within provision that is very specific to OH, adapting existing methods or tools to suit individual business is very common.

Audit is described as a cycle as it is a continual process. Building on the outline in Figure 10.1, there are many variations of the cycle, with four to seven steps outlined, depending on which method is considered. Figure 10.3 shows a generic basic five-step audit cycle. This can be used for auditing manufacturing process, clinical care and administrative process.

Stage 1: Planning

Stage 1 is the planning. This is ensuring that the business is clear what is to be audited – when, why and how. Then the preparation – ensuring that standards and procedures are in place for all processes/tasks undertaken and that individuals tasked with the audit are prepared for the task. It involves ensuring that all information (results of surveys, statistical breakdown of results) is available so that the audit can be a smooth process, and establishing who is undertaking the audit, that the person has the resources and is appropriate for this task. Also an essential part of this process, especially if this is a first audit, is preparation for change. It needs to be approached as a positive action rather than a fault-finding exercise.

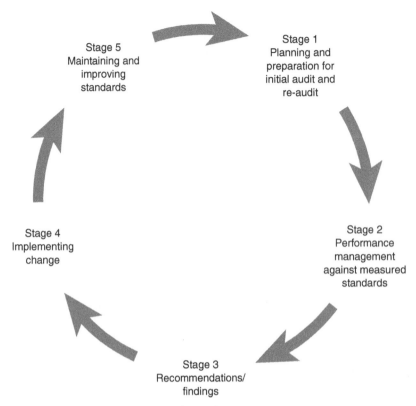

Figure 10.3 Basic five-step audit cycle

Stage 2: Performance management

In the second stage, the performance is measured against the standards – organisational standards, professional standards or statutory requirements. It is crucial to the quality element that the standards are appropriate to the service provided. It is also essential that the standards are measured in an appropriate way. This can range from tools from a checklist, to interview, to statistical analysis, feedback surveys or visual inspection. For those interested in methodology, there are many specific tools that can be found in audit and quality management reference books.

Stage 3: Recommendations/findings

This is where both areas of best practice, areas that require updating or areas requiring improvement can be identified and the plan for implementing this is established.

Stage 4: Implementing change

This needs to be approached as a positive outcome for best results as opposed to a negative criticism. Change is a continual process, especially in OH, so it is unlikely that any thorough audit will have no recommendations.

Stage 5: Sustaining standards and improvement

It is important that the audit and measure of quality outcome are not false – for example, everyone works to a particular standard over a short period of time to maximise audit results. The audit should be a valid and reliable measure of the quality of service offered. This stage is about ensuring motivation to sustain and improve standards is inherent within the service and participation in benchmarking.

It is unlikely that even a new OH business would have to start completely from scratch to write the standards and procedures that need to be in place to measure performance. Some structure can be put in place by following the professional and statutory requirements, then building on this to establish a tailored and effective audit system for the specific service.

One starting place is the *Small Business Guide*,[26] which gives an outline of the areas that need to be covered by standards and procedures. Although based in NHS practice and culture, the NICE *Principles for Best Practice in Clinical Audit* explains some of the philosophy behind culture change and maintaining clinical standards.[27] The SEQOHS published standards give another framework from which to work.[24] Various professional organisations, such as AOHNP (UK), have excellent member networking and information sharing and can be a useful source of guidance and advice.

Is the audit process research?

There has been much debate over the past two decades within healthcare (including the NHS) on whether clinical audit is in itself research. This is a complete topic within itself and more information can be found within Healthcare Quality Improvement Partnership,[28] NICE[29] and Health and Work Development Unit.[30]

To summarise what appears to be the current position of most significant bodies in this debate: clinical audit is not in itself necessarily research, but it does utilise research methodology in order to assess practice. Research questions can be answered by auditing information. For example, there is a whole body of potential research waiting to be undertaken within the valuable epidemiological data that OH organisations hold, where well-organised and thorough audit could be a valid methodology.

The audit cycle should aim to establish or highlight any gaps in evidence-based practice guidelines or standards – and this in itself should produce the impetus for research (Table 10.6).

Conclusion

Quality and audit within OH is a complex process with competing drivers and demands. It is an essential part of both the clinical and business side of OH and very worthwhile for both service quality and business/financial gains. Establishing and undertaking an effective process that is fit for the individual service is a challenge. It is also crucial to have an effective process in place so that benefits can be delivered and the process is neither time wasting nor a destructive process. As an individual practitioner, auditing

Table 10.6 Basic differences between research and (clinical) audit

Research	(Clinical) audit
Aims to establish best practice	Aims to evaluate how close practice is to defined standards and identify ways of improvement
Designed to be replicated and results generated beyond research group	Specific to area audited
Aims to generate or increase new knowledge	Aims to improve service and identify areas needing further knowledge
Is theory-driven	Is practice-based
(Dependent on design) but often one-off study	Ongoing, regular or continuous cycle

one's own professional practice is also an essential part of professional development, as outlined in Chapter 1, in addition to the revalidation of professional qualifications. There are many specific books and courses devoted to the subject of quality and audit, with differing methods of ensuring quality by general and specialist audit tools. For those interested in reading further, following the references cited and the business section of the local library are good starting points.

References

1 Black C (2008) *Working for a Healthier Tomorrow*. London: TSO, p. 16. Available online at: http://www.dwp.gov.uk/docs/hwwb-working-for-a-healthier-tomorrow.pdf (accessed 09.01.13).
2 WHO Europe (1999) *Guidelines on Quality Management in Multidisciplinary Occupational Health Services*. Copenhagen: WHO.
3 Hughes R, Higgenson I (2006) Discussion of quality and audit in health. *J Social Policy* 22 (1): 29–38.
4 Patel S (2010) Identifying best practice principles in audit of healthcare. *Nurs Stand* 24 (32): 40–48.
5 Burnett AC, Winyard G (1998) Clinical audit at the heart of clinical effectiveness. *J Clin Pract* 18 (1): 3–19.
6 Pursig RM (1999) *Zen and the Art of Motorcycle Maintenance: An inquiry into values*. London: Vintage.
7 Department of Health (1989) *Working for Patients*. White Paper. London: Department of Health.
8 Shaw C (1990) Criterion-based audit. *Br Med J* 300: 649. Available online at: http://www.bmj.com/content/300/6725/649 (accessed 13.7.13).
9 *Oxford Dictionary* (2012) Oxford: Oxford University Press.
10 Mech T, Young MD (2001) *VEMAs: Designing voluntary environmental management arrangements to improve natural resource management in agriculture and allied rural*

industries. Kingston, Australia: RIDC Publication. Available online at: www.myoung. net.au/water/publications/voluntary_environmental_CSL-15A.pdf (accessed 01.04.13).

11 Nightingale F (1860) *Notes on Nursing: What it is and what it is not.* New York: Appleton.

12 Department for Work and Pensions (2012) *Getting the Most Out of the Fit Note: Guidance for employers and line managers,* p. 10. Available online at: http://www.dwp. gov.uk/docs/fitnote-employers-linemanagers-guidance.pdf (accessed 02.04.13).

13 *Fitness for Work: The Government response to 'Health at Work – an Independent review of Sickness Absence'.* London: The Stationery Office. Available online at: http:// www.dwp.gov.uk/docs/health-at-work-gov-response.pdf.

14 Agius R (2006) *Seaton Practical Occupational Medicine.* London: Edward Arnold, p. 271.

15 www.nice.org.uk/nicemedia/pdf/bestpracticeclinicalaudit.pdf (accessed 01.04.13).

16 http://www.mohawk.nhshealthatwork.co.uk (accessed 01.04.13).

17 www.aohnp.co.uk.

18 www.bohrf.org.uk (accessed 01.04.13).

19 Nursing and Midwifery Council (2008) *The Code: Standards of conduct, performance and ethics for nurses and midwives.* London: NMC. Available online at: www.nmc-uk. org.

20 Parmenter D (2012) *Key Performance Indicators: Developing, implementing and using winning KPIs,* 2nd edn. Hoboken, NJ: John Wiley, p. 10.

21 Agius RM, Lee RJ, Murdoch RM, Symington IS, Riddle HFV, Seaton A (1993) Occupational physicians and their work: Prospects for audit. *Occup Med* 43: 159–163.

22 Agius R (undated) *Correspondence Assessment/Audit Tool in/for Occupational Health (CATOH).* Available online at: www.agius.com/hew/audit/catoh.htm.

23 Agius RM, Seaton A, Lee RJ (1994) An audit of occupational health consultation records. *Occup Med* 44 (3): 151–167.

24 www.seqohs.org.

25 Oakley K (2008) *Occupational Health Nursing.* Oxford: Wiley, pp. 87–103.

26 http://www.thecqi.org/Documents/knowledge/small_business_standard.pdf (accessed 01.04.13).

27 NICE (2002) *Principles for Best Practice in Clinical Audit.* Oxford: Radcliffe Medical Press. Available online at: www.nice.org.uk/media/796/23/bestpracticeclinicalaudit.pdf.

28 www.hqip.org.uk.

29 www.nice.org.uk.

30 www.rcplondon.ac.uk/rcp/clinical-standards-department/health-and-work-development-unit.

Appendix: additional resources

Teresa Harrison and Jeremy Smith

The following resources relate to Chapters 1–5

http://aeromedical.org/List: aviation medicine

http://health.groups.yahoo.com/group/globalocchyg-list: industrial hygiene

http://list.uvm.edu/archives/safety.html: safety

http://subscribe.occhealthnews.net: occupational and environmental medicine

http://thorax.bmj.com/content/63/3/240.full: standards of care for occupational asthma

http://www.absa.org/resgroups.html: bio safety

http://www.bohrf.org.uk/downloads/OA_Guide-1.pdf: occupational asthma guide for occupational healthcare professionals

http://www.bohrf.org.uk/downloads/OCDU_Guide-1.pdf: occupational contact dermatitis and urticaria guide for occupational health professionals

http://www.bohrf.org.uk/downloads/Work_and_the_Menopause-A_Guide_for_Managers.pdf: leaflet advising managers on the research undertaken on women at work and http://www.fitfortravel.nhs.uk/destinations.aspxhe menopause

http://www.ccohs.ca/hscanada/hscsubscribe.html: Canadian Centre for Occupational Health and Safety

http://www.dwp.gov.uk/health-work-and-well-being/our-work/oh-adviceline/: general advice for small- to medium-sized businesses

http://www.dwp.gov.uk/health-work-and-well-being/our-work/workplace-well-being-tool/: workplace wellbeing tool designed to help employers improve the health and wellbeing of people in their organisation

http://www.fom.ac.uk/health-at-work-2/advice-for-people-with-disabilities: advice for individuals with disabilities

https://www.gov.uk/government/publications/at-a-glance: up-to-date Driver and Vehicle Licensing Agency medical guidance re class 1 and 2 drivers

http://www.hse.gov.uk/health-surveillance: information for employers regarding health surveillance and what their responsibilities are

http://www.llttf.com/: Living Life to the Full website that gives help and advice on people suffering from mental health problems

http://www.macmillan.org.uk/Home.aspx: offers advice for both patients and health professionals about cancer and work

http://www.ncbi.nlm.nih.gov/pubmed/23374107: UK standards of care for occupational contact dermatitis and occupational contact urticaria.

http://www.nhs.uk/LiveWell/Workplacehealth/Pages/workplacehome.aspx: general guidance on workplace health

http://www.occupationalasthma.com

http://www.rcog.org.uk/recovering-well: patient information on recovery following gynae-cological surgery

http://www.rcplondon.ac.uk/resources/upper-limb-disorders-guideline: upper-limb guidance produced by the Royal College of Physicians

http://www.rcseng.ac.uk/patients/get-well-soon/arthroscopic-meniscectomy: patient infor-mation for anyone who is recovering from, or is about to undergo, surgery to have a torn meniscus dealt with by keyhole or arthroscopic surgery

http://www.workingfit.com/Surgery/FitnessSurgery.html: a general guide to fitness follow-ing surgery, some evidenced

https://moodgym.anu.edu.au/welcome: a free self-help program to teach cognitive behav-iour therapy skills to people vulnerable to depression and anxiety

https://www.hse.gov.uk/forms/health/emasoffices.htm: list of regional offices and contact numbers for Employment Medical Advisory Service, also provides the links for the forms related to the work of HSE-appointed doctors and approved medical examiners of divers (AMEDs)

https://www.tuc.org.uk/publications/index.cfm: Trades Union Congress has several publi-cations around work and health

www.fitfortravel.nhs.uk: travel advice from the NHS

www.hse.gov.uk/statistics: up-to-date information on health and safety statistics

www.vtstutorials.co.uk: a website of free tutorials, one being internet research skills

Carter T (2006) *Fitness to Drive: A guide for health professionals.* London: Royal Society of Medicine Press.

Gillen T (2002) *Leadership Skills for Boosting Performance.* London: CIPD.

Hogarth J, Khan S (2004) *Fit for Work: The complete guide to managing sickness absence and rehabilitation.* London: EEF The Manufacturers Organisation.

Miller D, Lipsedge M, Litchfield P (2002) *Work and Mental Health . . . An employer's guide.* London: Gaskell.

The following resources relate to Chapter 6

http://bma.org.uk/practical-support-at-work/contracts/occupational-health: this guide pro-vides up-to-date information on all aspects of occupational health, including an explana-tion of the expected duties of occupational physicians and practical advice on specific aspects of the role, such as conducting health assessments and providing advice on sick-ness absence

http://www.health4work.nhs.uk/occupational_health_services?gclid=CJHo64v1rrcCFVD MtAoddl4A4Q: Health for Work Adviceline

http://www.hse.gov.uk/index.htm: guidance on statutory requirements for health assessment

Beaumont DG (2003) The interaction between general practitioners and occupational health professionals in relation to rehabilitation for work: A Delphi study. *Occup Med* 53: 249–253.

Ferguson GT, Enright PL, Buist AS, Higgins MW (2000) Office spirometry for lung health assessment in adults: A consensus statement from the National Lung Health Education Program. *Chest* 117 (4): 1146–1161.

Feuerstein M, Huang GD, Ortiz JM, Shaw WS, Miller VI, Wood PM, Cohn S (2003) Integrated case management for work-related upper-extremity disorders: Impact of patient satisfac-tion on health and work status. *J Occup Environment Med* 45 (8): 803–812.

Kanter J (1989) Clinical case management: Definition, principles, components. *Hosp Commun Psychiatry* 40: 361–368.

Stucki G (2005) International Classification of Functioning, Disability, and Health (ICF): A promising framework and classification for rehabilitation medicine. *Am J Phys Med Rehabil* 84: 733–740.

Stucki G, Ewert T, Cieza A (2002) Value and application of the ICF in rehabilitation medicine. *Disabil Rehabil* 20: 932–938.

Waddell G, Burton AK (2001) Occupational health guidelines for the management of low back pain at work: Evidence review. *Occup Med* 51: 124–135.

The following resources relate to Chapter 7

http://www.bohrf.org.uk/downloads/cmh_hp.pdf: workplace interventions for people with common mental health problems: a summary for health professionals

http://www.cipd.co.uk/binaries/5715MentalHealthguideWEB.pdf: developed by Mind and the Chartered Institute of Personnel and Development, this guidance contains information, practical advice and templates to help managers facilitate conversations about stress and mental health problems and put in place support so employees can stay well and in work.

http://www.hse.gov.uk/stress/furtheradvice/stressandmentalhealth.htm: line managers' competency tool. It allows managers to reflect upon whether or not their management style is having a negative impact

http://www.hse.gov.uk/stress/pdfs/returntowork.pdf: useful tool for employee and manager to discuss the impact of work stressors and possible accommodations

http://www.hse.gov.uk/stress/standards/pdfs/indicatortool.pdf: Health and Safety Executive management standards indicator tool allows individuals to identify possible work stressors

http://www.llttf.com/: Living Life to the Full – online cognitive behavioural therapy

http://www.mindfulemployer.net/MINDFUL%20EMPLOYER%20Line%20Managers%20Resource.pdf: downloadable PDF resource for employers

www.hse.gov.uk/stress/furtheradvice/stressandmentalhealth: Health and Safety Executive guidance on stress at work and mental health

www.mind.org.uk: 'We're here to make sure anyone with a mental health problem has somewhere to turn for advice and support'

www.shaw-trust.org.uk: Shaw Trust is a not-for-profit organisation helping disabled people or those at disadvantage to find and sustain employment or enjoy more independent living

The following resources relate to Chapter 8

http://www.cbhscheme.com: Constructing Better Health is responsible for delivering the national scheme for the management of occupational health in the construction industry

http://www.peoplealchemy.co.uk: alchemy is a comprehensive online resource of management tools, tips, methods and practical information.

Association of Occupational Health Nurse Practitioners (UK) (1998) *Information for Independent Occupational Health Practice*. Peterhead, Aberdeenshire: AOHNP(UK).

Association of Occupational Health Nurse Practitioners (UK) (2008) *Running an Occupational Health Business*. Peterhead, Aberdeenshire: AOHNP(UK).

Snashall D, Patel D (2012) *ABC of Occupational and Environmental Medicine,* 3rd edn. Chichester: Wiley-Blackwell.

Westerholm P, Nilstun T, Øvretveit J (eds) (2004) *Practical Ethics in Occupational Health*. Oxford: Radcliffe Medical Press.

The following resources relate to Chapter 9

http://www.beds.ac.uk/research/ihr/statistics-and-epidemiology-group: the Statistics and Epidemiology Group is part of the Institute for Health Research, focusing on the application of methodology for the evaluation of health interventions and chronic disease epidemiology

http://www.bmj.com/: *British Medical Journal*

www.epiresearch.org: the Society for Epidemiologic Research was created in 1967 with the purpose of engaging students and new researchers with senior faculty in a meaningful way

www.kingsfund.org.uk: the King's Fund is an independent charity working to improve health and healthcare in England. 'We help to shape policy and practice through research and analysis; develop individuals, teams and organisations; promote understanding of the health and social care system; and bring people together to learn, share knowledge and debate'

www.lshtm.ac.uk: this course aims to equip students with the knowledge and skills to make valuable contributions to both epidemiological research and public health

www.ucl.ac.uk/epidemiology: a multidisciplinary department located in Central London. Staff aim to develop a better understanding of health and prevention of ill health through vigorous research and the development of research methodology

www.wellcome.ac.uk: the Wellcome Trust has been working with a variety of partners to support data sharing among epidemiological and public health researchers

The following resources relate to Chapter 10

http://www.acsregistrars.com/: ACS Registrars is regarded as being one of the premier ISO 9001, ISO 14001, ISO 27001, OHSAS 18001 and PAS 43 (NHSS 17 & 17b) registration/certification bodies

http://www.bsigroup.co.uk: 'We were the world's first national standards body and we remain a leading global standards maker. We are the UK's National Standards Body, representing UK interests worldwide'

http://www.cqc.org.uk: Care Quality Commission

http://www.gmc-uk.org: General Medical Council

http://www.nhsemployers.org/Aboutus/Publications/Documents/Occupational%20 health%20and%20safety%20standards.pdf: these initiatives have now been built upon by the publication of Dr Steven Boorman's NHS Health and Well-being Review, published in August and October 2009

http://www.nice.org.uk/guidance/qualitystandards/QualityStandardsLibrary.jsp: National Institute for Health and Care Exellence quality standards topic library

http://www.nmc-uk.org: Nursing and Midwifery Council

http://www.qaa.ac.uk: 'We are the Quality Assurance Agency for Higher Education (QAA). Our mission is to safeguard standards and improve the quality of UK higher education'

http://www.rcplondon.ac.uk: 'In keeping with our commitment to improving healthcare and the health of the population, we lead on and collaborate with partners on a range of projects and programmes of activities to support physicians, promote patient-centred care, and improve standards of clinical practice and public health'

http://www.rcuk.ac.uk: Research Councils UK is responsible for investing public money in research in the UK to advance knowledge and generate new ideas which lead to a productive economy and healthy society and contribute to a sustainable world

http://www.ssiacymru.org.uk: these pages have been developed to promote best practice and to provide support to those working within quality assurance

www.adamasconsulting.com: independent clinical quality assurance consultancy specialising in worldwide clinical research audit and clinical quality management

www.gov.uk/government/organisations/department-of-health

Patel S (2010) Achieving quality assurance through clinical audit. *Nurs Manage* 17 (3): 28–34.

Index